A USML

MW01591361

Psychiatry

10th Edition

A USMLE STEP 2 REVIEW

Psychiatry

10th Edition

700

Questions & Answers

Edited by

Carlyle H. Chan, MD
*Associate Professor
and Director, Residency Education*

Harry Prosen, MD
*Professor and Chairman
Department of Psychiatry
and Behavioral Medicine
Medical College of Wisconsin
Milwaukee, Wisconsin*

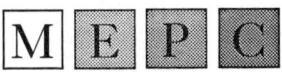

Medical Examination
Publishing Company

APPLETON & LANGE
Norwalk, Connecticut

Notice: The authors and the publisher of this volume have taken care to make certain that the doses of drugs and schedules of treatment are correct and compatible with the standards generally accepted at the time of publication. Nevertheless, as new information becomes available, changes in treatment and in the use of drugs become necessary. The reader is advised to carefully consult the instruction and information material included in the package insert of each drug or therapeutic agent before administration. This advice is especially important when using new or infrequently used drugs. The publisher disclaims any liability, loss, injury, or damage incurred as a consequence, directly or indirectly, or the use and application of any of the contents of the volume.

95 96 97 98 / 10 9 8 7 6 5 4 3 2 1

Prentice Hall International (UK) Limited, *London*
Prentice Hall of Australia Pty. Limited, *Sydney*
Prentice Hall Canada, Inc., *Toronto*
Prentice Hall Hispanoamericana, S.A., *Mexico*
Prentice Hall of India Private Limited, *New Delhi*
Prentice Hall of Japan, Inc., *Tokyo*
Simon & Schuster Asia Pte. Ltd., *Singapore*
Editora Prentice Hall do Brasil Ltda., *Rio de Janeiro*
Prentice Hall, *Englewood Cliffs, New Jersey*

ISBN 0-8385-5780-5

90000

ISBN: 0-8385-5780-5
ISSN: 1080-7985

9 780838 557808

Acquisitions Editor: Jamie Mount Kircher
Production Services: Rainbow Graphics, Inc.

PRINTED IN THE UNITED STATES OF AMERICA

List of Contributors

Elizabeth Caspary, MD, Assistant Professor, Department of Psychiatry and Behavioral Medicine, Medical College of Wisconsin, Milwaukee

Carlyle H. Chan, MD, Associate Professor and Director, Residency Education, Department of Psychiatry and Behavioral Medicine, Medical College of Wisconsin, Milwaukee

Robert Chayer, MD, Child Psychiatry Fellow, Department of Psychiatry and Behavioral Medicine, Medical College of Wisconsin, Milwaukee

Kathryn C. Krieg, MD, Assistant Professor, Department of Psychiatry and Behavioral Medicine, Medical College of Wisconsin, Milwaukee

Gunnar Larson, MD, Assistant Professor, Department of Psychiatry and Behavioral Medicine, Medical College of Wisconsin, Milwaukee

Joseph B. Layde, MD, JD, Assistant Professor, Department of Psychiatry and Behavioral Medicine, Medical College of Wisconsin, Milwaukee; Medical Program Director, Acute Care Inpatient Services, Milwaukee County Mental Health Complex

John E. Pappenheim, MD, Assistant Professor, Department of Psychiatry and Behavioral Medicine, Medical College of Wisconsin, Milwaukee; Director of Neuropsychiatric Services, Columbia Hospital, Milwaukee

Harry Prosen, MD, Professor and Chairman, Department of Psychiatry and Behavioral Medicine, Medical College of Wisconsin, Milwaukee

Contents

Preface

The tenth edition of *Medical Examination Review: Psychiatry* has been revised and updated to keep in step with current trends in medical education and the continuing explosion of scientific knowledge. Featuring a total of 700 questions with explanatory answers, the book is designed to help you review your course work and prepare for the United States Medical Licensing Examination Step 2.

The range of subjects included in this book is based on the content outline of the National Board of Medical Examiners, which develops the question pool for the test mentioned above, and reflects the scope and depth of what is taught in medical schools today. The questions were carefully selected to enhance the review process by challenging the reader's problem-solving abilities and grasp of underlying principles.

A final chapter on case studies provides a comprehensive review of clinical situations in psychiatry. Questions based on each of the subject areas covered in the book are presented in a manner more closely simulating the actual examination experience. Using this book, you may identify areas of strength and weakness in your own command of the subject. Specific references to widely used textbooks allow you to return to the authoritative source for further study.

The Editors wish to gratefully acknowledge Shawna Elliot, Lisa Loerzel, and Donna Bova for their contributions in preparing this manuscript.

A USMLE STEP 2 REVIEW

Psychiatry

10th Edition

1

Basic Principles: Growth, Development, Psychodynamics, and Personality Theory

Robert Chayer

DIRECTIONS (Questions 1 through 37): Each of the questions or incomplete statements below is followed by five suggested answers or completions. Select the ONE that is best in each case.

---

1. Temperamental attributes that describe the behavioral *style* of children include
   A. verbal loquaciousness
   B. adaptability to new situations
   C. physical strength
   D. harshness of affective response
   E. guilt in the face of discipline

2. Stranger anxiety, evidence of the development of a strong attachment bond, usually appears by
   A. the first week of life
   B. 4 to 6 weeks, in association with the "biological" smile
   C. three months, with the appearance of the "social" smile
   D. 7 to 8 months, when the child has some capacity for mental representation
   E. one year, when the child can move away from the stranger effectively

3. Bowlby described the sequential pattern of *protest, despair,* and *detachment* as the infant's response to
   A. human contact after cocaine exposure in utero
   B. neglect by the caretaker
   C. sensory overload
   D. separation from the major caretaker
   E. physical abuse

4. In learning theory, positive reinforcement(s)
   A. does not change effectiveness by the scheduling of the reinforcement
   B. diminishes the response
   C. is an inherent characteristic of many drugs of abuse
   D. usually is ineffective
   E. works best with children

5. All of the following statements are true of social–cognitive learning theory EXCEPT
   A. cognitive processes are viewed as important parts of the *reinforcement* paradigm
   B. reinforcers with *less* information are more powerful
   C. goal setting and self-instruction gain strength through *feedback*
   D. *expectancies* develop quickly about outcome with self-observation
   E. *modeling* by the observation of others can be effective in both children and adults

6. In Piaget's theoretical framework, cognitive development is completed when the child reaches
   A. the sensorimotor phase
   B. cause and effect thinking
   C. the formal (abstract) phase
   D. concrete operational thinking
   E. the preoperational (symbolic) phase

7. Piaget's stage of development usually linked with the "latency" phase in psychosexual development is
   A. the sensorimotor stage
   B. formal operations
   C. preoperational thought
   D. logical thought
   E. concrete operations

8. The personality theory of Carl Jung includes all of the following features EXCEPT
   A. there is no *unconscious,* as all mental activity is available to use
   B. mental activity is built around *complexes,* groups of ideas associated with emotionally toned events
   C. *archetypes,* systems of readiness to respond to emotional cues, are inherited with brain structure
   D. *individuation* is a major developmental task of adult life
   E. *neurosis* results from the influence of complexes

9. Attainment of Piaget's concrete operations stage in cognitive development requires
   A. the ability to reason about reasoning
   B. the ability to grasp probability
   C. the capability to think about one's thoughts
   D. adolescence
   E. the concept of conservation of physical characteristics

10. Which of the following steps in language development is out of temporal order?
    A. use of interaction to signal stress
    B. identifying objects by pointing
    C. use of simple sentences
    D. counting serially to ten
    E. attaining a vocabulary of 500 words

11. Waking electroencephalographic (EEG) patterns follow usual developmental patterns. Which feature below is mismatched?
    A. gradual increase in slow frequencies in the first year of life
    B. increasing proportion of alpha frequencies (8 to 13 cycles per second) in mid-childhood
    C. delta frequencies predominant in adolescence
    D. suppression of alpha with mental activity
    E. symmetrical beta/fast activities in adult anterior brain regions

12. This principle maintains that, to assure full and healthy development, critical tasks of each developmental period must be mastered at the proper time and in sequence. It is known as
    A. epigenesis
    B. progression
    C. regression
    D. development
    E. maturation

13. In Freudian theory, the investment of psychic/emotional energy in a mental representation is known as
    A. part object
    B. libido
    C. cathexis
    D. structure
    E. drive

14. Normally, the oedipal stage in psychosexual development is *resolved* by
    A. identification with the parent of the opposite sex
    B. identification with the parent of the same sex
    C. projection of sexualized feelings to peers

    D. regression to a pre-oedipal position

    E. fixation on the opposite sex parent

15. All of the following statements about the superego, in psychosexual development, are accurate EXCEPT
    - **A.** it is derived through identification with parents and their substitutes
    - **B.** it contains the conscience
    - **C.** it is initially rigid and punitive
    - **D.** it must be in place before entry into the oedipal period
    - **E.** as children mature, their early superego absolutes are modified

16. Undoing, as a neurotic defense
    - **A.** allows separation of affect and impulse from idea
    - **B.** requires an act to prevent the consequences of the thought or impulse
    - **C.** sets up character patterns that are exactly the opposite of the underlying impulse
    - **D.** externalizes the impulse to another
    - **E.** shifts the focus of the impulse to a different, more acceptable, act or thought

17. A term referring to the ego's anticipation of the experience of danger is
    - **A.** signal anxiety
    - **B.** castration anxiety
    - **C.** separation anxiety
    - **D.** id anxiety
    - **E.** performance anxiety

18. The fearful anticipation of the loss of an important relationship is called
    - **A.** signal anxiety
    - **B.** castration anxiety
    - **C.** separation anxiety
    - **D.** id anxiety
    - **E.** performance anxiety

19. Mahler called the stage in which the child becomes aware of being separate from the mother and able to relate to a variety of objects/persons the

   A. autistic phase
   B. symbiotic phase
   C. separation–individuation phase
   D. oedipal phase
   E. rapprochement crisis

20. Normal rapprochement, in Mahler's theory, has all of the following features EXCEPT

   A. targeted behavior occurs between 16 and 24 months
   B. it depends on the cognitive awareness of separateness from the parent
   C. ambivalence and ambitendency are the hallmarks
   D. it is marked by the beginning of greater interest in the world
   E. it parallels the anal and early oedipal psychosexual stages of development

21. The anal phase of psychosexual development occurs

   A. between 18 and 36 months
   B. in conjunction with superego guilt over pleasurable bowel function
   C. in response to weaning from the breast
   D. when parents start toileting too early
   E. without a clear erotic "zone"

22. Superego anxiety, in psychoanalytic theory

   A. occurs when a person feels he will lose control of his impulses
   B. arises from the anticipation of discovery and the subsequent guilt
   C. has as its hallmark fantasies of genital mutilation
   D. is associated with the emergence of the awareness of rage
   E. is commonly seen in homosexual panic

23. Splitting, a feature of early development and prominent in some pathological conditions, is a

   A. primitive idealization
   B. projective identification
   C. form of identification

D. lack of integration
E. regression to impulsivity

24. Late childhood, from ages 6 to 10, generally is characterized by all of the following EXCEPT
  A. increased influence of the extrafamily group
  B. the development of formal thought (Piaget)
  C. a growing sense of industry or inferiority
  D. learning of the customs of the society
  E. less marked sexual changes than during stages pre- or post-

25. Which of the following is NOT an ego function?
  A. motor capacity
  B. reality testing
  C. defense mechanisms
  D. instinctual drives
  E. self and object representation

26. The anal stage of psychosexual development
  A. is culturally determined
  B. occurs in the third year of life
  C. is a psychic organization period related to traits of cleanliness in later life
  D. leads to identification with the same sex parent
  E. is crucial to the formation of basic trust in the child's personality

27. Which of the following statements is NOT true?
  A. Piaget's theory of cognitive development calls for a constant reorganization of cognitive capabilities
  B. by the seventh or eighth month, infants reared in well-supported environments develop a wariness about contact with strangers
  C. at the seventh to eighth month, infants gain an idea of an object separate from their sensory motor pattern of involvement with the object
  D. Kohut's developmental lines parallel those of Freud's theory
  E. "separation" concerns the child's disengagement from the mother

28. The personality theory of Melanie Klein
   A. recognizes splitting only later in development as a child develops the ability to express good and bad through language
   B. focuses on early object relations as a cornerstone of development
   C. argues for superego development in association with oedipal trauma in middle childhood
   D. requires very slow-going treatment, with early reality-based interpretations around the relationship with the therapist
   E. delays negative transference interpretations until a good deal of education about therapy has been obtained

29. Mahler's theory of object relations presents which of the following as characteristic of the first months of life (the autistic phase)?
   A. there is a clear distinction by the infant between internal and external
   B. the predominant feeling state of the infant is one of self-absorbed pleasure
   C. the infant is critically aware of the mother's caretaking
   D. the infant must fight the intrusion of external stimuli
   E. the infant–mother link is fragile and easily disrupted by other caretakers, including the father

30. The psychoanalytic theory of depression emphasizes all of the following EXCEPT
   A. actual or fantasized interpersonal loss
   B. a breakdown in regulation of self-esteem
   C. aggression turned inward toward the self
   D. splitting of "all good" from "all bad" parts of the self
   E. an intersystemic conflict between the superego and id

31. Psychoanalytic theory posits that sadomasochistic sexuality has its core developmentally in
   A. oedipal phase disappointments in the dominant (ie, sadistic) parent
   B. lifelong distress caused by early weaning from the bitten breast of the mother
   C. the anal sadistic phase of childhood
   D. brutal interaction during early adolescent heterosexual experimentation

E. an early separation of libidinal and aggressive drives, such that a dramatic increase in "pain" is required to elicit pleasurable sensations

32. Early adolescent development, as a phase, includes all of the following features EXCEPT
   A. the onset of puberty
   B. the average male is ahead of the average female in physical growth at the same age
   C. an increase in sexual preoccupation
   D. a turning away from the parents to peers
   E. repressed oedipal wishes gaining strength

33. The psychological development of children in foster care
   A. will parallel that of those adopted early
   B. usually is not influenced by the age of placement
   C. usually shows a lack of attachment to natural parents after a short time
   D. generally is worse than the development of same aged children placed in institutional (eg, orphanage) care
   E. when studied appropriately, can be a useful research tool to judge the transmission of psychiatric disorders

34. Which of the following statements is true concerning acquired immune deficiency syndrome (AIDS) in childhood?
   A. generally it is not a fatal disorder
   B. it will present, eventually, in close to 100% of those infants born to human immunodeficiency virus (HIV)-infected women
   C. it includes, as a significant portion of the total, children who acquired blood/blood product-borne infection (eg, hemophilia and sickle cell patients)
   D. it frequently will require placement of the child with alternate caretakers
   E. affected children usually are quite different from children with other chronic illness

35. Attachment by an infant to a caretaking figure requires
  A. a mentally healthy caretaker
  B. consistent interaction with the caretaking person
  C. lack of abuse by the caretaker
  D. the child's ability to hear
  E. contact beginning in the infant's "sensitive" period in the immediate postdelivery period

36. In classical psychoanalytic theory, an instinctual drive is characterized as having all of the features below EXCEPT
  A. a specific pattern
  B. a source
  C. an object
  D. an aim
  E. an intensity

37. "Primary process" thinking
  A. uses logic
  B. is most prominent in adolescence
  C. is primitive, dominated by emotion
  D. has the capacity for delay and modulation
  E. takes into consideration the external reality

DIRECTIONS (Questions 38 through 105): Each group of questions below consists of lettered headings followed by a list of numbered words, phrases, or statements. For each numbered word, phrase, or statement, select the ONE lettered heading that is most closely associated with it. Each lettered heading may be selected once, more than once, or not at all.

Questions 38 through 42

    A. homeostasis (0 to 3 months)
    B. attachment (2 to 7 months)
    C. somatopsychological differentiation (3 to 10 months)
    D. behavioral organization, initiative, and internalization (9 to 24 months)
    E. representational capacity, differentiation, and consolidation (18 to 48 months)

38. Imitative learning is the dominant form

39. The process can be distorted if the caretaker responds in a mechanical manner

40. Use of the primary senses (ie, sight, smell, touch) is the predominant mode of interaction

41. Pretend play and symbolism emerge

42. Pathological autistic (Diagnostic and Statistical Manual–4th Edition [DSM–IV]) patterns can become evident

Questions 43 through 46

    A. fetal alcohol syndrome
    B. fetal hydantoin syndrome
    C. both A and B
    D. neither A nor B

43. Microcephaly

44. Mental retardation

45. Short stature

46. Genetic transmission

Questions 47 through 50

    A. screen memory
    B. amnesia
    C. both A and B
    D. neither A nor B

47. May be psychogenic or from organic injury

48. May precede or postdate the event which is its focus

49. May be expressed as the family romance fantasy

50. May be analyzable

Questions 51 through 53

    A. affect
    B. mood
    C. both A and B
    D. neither A nor B

51. Outwardly observable

52. Subjectively experienced

53. Relatively stable and long-lasting state

Questions 54 through 57

    A. anxiety dreams
    B. night terrors
    C. both A and B
    D. neither A nor B

54. Stage IV arousal phenomena

55. Not remembered

56. Occur in young children

57. A sign of psychopathology

Questions 58 through 61

    A. early adolescence
    B. mid-adolescence
    C. late adolescence

58. Moves away from bodily preoccupation

59. Uses solid skills in abstract thinking to address real-life problems

60. Exhibits normative rebellious behavior (eg, dress, hairstyle)

61. Sexuality is repressed and denied

Questions 62 through 65

    A. young adulthood
    B. middle adulthood
    C. late adulthood

62. Expansion of concerns beyond egotistical focus

63. Establishment of firm sense of social/sexual self

64. Generativity is an underlying theme

65. Less social posturing ("This is me, take it or leave it")

Questions 66 through 69

    A. dynamic hypothesis
    B. economic hypothesis
    C. topographic hypothesis
    D. genetic hypothesis
    E. structural hypothesis

66. Consists of three functional systems: id, ego, and superego

67. Expresses in quantitative terms the outcome of intrapsychic conflict

68. Addresses the conflict between drives and defenses

69. Consists of three systems: conscious, preconscious, and unconscious

Questions 70 through 74

    A. oral period
    B. anal period
    C. genital period
    D. latency period
    E. adolescence

70. Shame may be a component

71. Sexual curiosity is limited

72. The Oedipus complex develops

73. Dependency is a characteristic

74. Castration anxiety is highlighted

Questions 75 through 78

    A. undoing
    B. turning against the self
    C. denial
    D. rationalization
    E. identification

75. A child believes his deceased sibling is away

76. Pornography is studied "scientifically"

77. A boy insists on taking his father's pen to school

78. Sins are confessed before a group

Questions 79 through 83

    A. denial
    B. projection
    C. repression
    D. displacement
    E. rationalization

79. Impulses are banished from consciousness

80. Plausible motives are substituted to mask real ones

81. Thoughts that are consciously not able to be tolerated are ignored

82. Others are seen to have the person's desires

83. Anger at the employer is directed at the spouse

Questions 84 through 88

    A. sublimination
    B. conversion
    C. introjection
    D. dissociation
    E. reaction formation

84. Drives are directed to socially accepted channels

85. Unconscious urges are expressed by character traits that are the opposite of those expected

86. There are special sensory or peripheral nervous system symptoms in the face of anxiety-producing conflict

87. The features of another's personality are apparent in one's own ego structure

88. Behaviors and feelings are separated from normal consciousness and control, with accompanying amnesia

Questions 89 through 91

    A. family romance
    B. primal scene
    C. oedipal victor
    D. imaginary companion

89. A boy announces he will marry his mother "when I get big"

90. A girl tells her friends, "My real parents are just having me stay here"

91. A boy tells the teacher his mother and father "fight in bed"

Questions 92 through 94

    A. differentiation subphase
    B. practicing subphase
    C. rapprochement subphase
    D. on the way to object constancy

92. Toddler uses mother to move large toy, never finding her placement "correct"

93. Toddler explores the environment while using mother's lap as a storage place for toys

94. Toddler calms when hearing mother's voice from another room

Questions 95 through 97

    A. oral stage
    B. anal stage
    C. separation–individuation stage
    D. phallic–oedipal stage
    E. latency stage

95. Problems trusting in the reliability of others

96. Problems with doubt about skills

97. Problems with initiative about tasks

Questions 98 through 101

    A. oral phase of psychosexual development
    B. anal phase of psychosexual development
    C. phallic phase of psychosexual development
    D. none of the above

98. Erikson's stage of initiative versus guilt

99. Erikson's stage of autonomy versus shame and doubt

100. Erikson's stage of industry versus inferiority

101. Erikson's stage of identity versus role diffusion

Questions 102 through 105

    A. Turner syndrome
    B. Down syndrome
    C. Klinefelter syndrome
    D. Fragile X (Fra-X) syndrome
    E. Prader–Willi syndrome

102. No clear genetic pattern

103. A nonsex chromosome abnormality

104. An X chromosome pattern

105. An abnormal chromosome pattern, evident only with special culture technique

Basic Principles: Growth, Development, Psychodynamics, and Personality Theory

Explanatory Answers

1. (B) Temperamental attributes are the "how" of behavior rather than the "why" or "what." Adaptability to new situations is a prime example of such a trait. (**Ref. 1,** p. 43)

2. (D) Stranger anxiety typically is stronger toward totally unknown persons than more familiar ones. Autistic children lack this developmental marker. (**Ref. 1,** p. 43)

3. (D) The response to separation from the major caretaker is felt by Bowlby and other attachment theorists to be similar to that of the adult mourning after the loss to death of a loved person. Bowlby believed that the sequence of protest, despair, and detachment involves ambivalent feelings towards the caregiver, both wanting the caregiver and becoming angry because of being deserted. Attachment disorders can result in failure-to-thrive syndromes, psychosocial dwarfism, separation anxiety disorder, avoidant personality disorder, depressive disorders, delinquency, academic problems, and borderline intelligence. (**Ref. 1,** p. 164)

4. (C) Drugs of abuse are highly sought by both animals and humans; they are powerful reinforcers at the biological level. Positive reinforcement is the process by which certain consequences of a response increase the probability that the response will occur again. (**Ref. 1,** p. 167)

5. (B) The key to social cognitive learning theory is that *more* information leads to more effective and predictable outcomes. Modeling, goal-setting, and self-instruction are all designed to create expectancies of learning situations. (**Ref. 9,** p. 268)

6. (C) Abstract thinking is the pinnacle of Piaget's theoretical constructs. The ability to think in a formal, highly logical, systematic, and symbolic manner is usually obtained from the age of 11 to the end of adolescence. Many impaired individuals never reach it. (**Ref. 1,** p. 159)

7. (E) Latency is the period in psychodynamic theory that occurs prior to the onset of puberty and adolescence. This time period would coincide with Piaget's stage of concrete operations, which occurs between ages 7 and 11. This period is marked by a focus on the concrete, real, and perceivable world of objects and events. It features the emergence of logical (cause–effect) reasoning and the ability to sequence and serialize. The child begins to appreciate another's point of view. (**Ref. 1,** pp. 20–23, 262)

8. (A) Jung's theory contains a major role for the unconscious, with both a *personal* unconscious (related to complexes), and a *collective* unconscious (related to inherited archetypes). The concept of the collective unconscious was one area where Jung diverged from Freud's ideas after initially being a disciple. (**Ref. 1,** p. 256)

9. (E) Length, mass, weight, and volume are the primary working concepts that Piaget studied in children in the concrete operations stage of cognitive development. Children in this stage use these concepts to order and group things in their environment. (**Ref. 1,** p. 159)

10. **(D)** Children usually count serially to ten by the age of five years. All the other skills are in place by age 36 months. (**Ref. 1,** pp. 41–42)

11. **(C)** Delta frequencies are defined as slower than 4 cycles per second and is generally associated with stage 3 and 4 of sleep, with more than 60% of stage 4 sleep being delta frequency in the adult. Delta frequencies are abnormal in the waking state in all age groups. (**Ref. 9,** pp. 157–158)

12. **(A)** Epigenesis is a principle adopted from embryology. It is most strongly associated with Erikson's theories of development. (**Ref. 1,** p. 157)

13. **(C)** Cathexis is a metaphorical concept derived from a Greek word substituting for an untranslatable concept from Freud's original German. It may have little relationship to the *actual* person or thing and is flexible in form—ie, cathexis can be increased or withdrawn. (**Ref. 1,** p. 241)

14. **(B)** Oedipal resolution normally allows settling of sexual tension by identification with the same sex parent in an unconflicted fashion. Until this resolution, the theory suggests a conflict with the same sex parent for the attention of the opposite sex parent. (**Ref. 1,** p. 46)

15. **(D)** The superego, classically described as the seat of the conscience and the focus of most neurotic pathology, is not formed until the Oedipus complex is resolved. The superego initially is the internalization of parental standards and values that includes the ego-ideal (what one should do) and moral conscience (what one should not do). (**Ref. 1,** p. 248)

16. **(B)** Undoing is felt to be a key defense in the psychoanalytic understanding of the obsessive–compulsive mechanisms of everyday life, especially in children and their games. Additionally, learning theory suggests that anxiety reduction of feelings attached to an obsessional thought are the motivation for compulsive behaviors. (**Ref. 1,** p. 600)

17. **(A)** Signal anxiety may be produced at the subconscious or unconscious level. It calls the ego to mobilize protective measures when the "danger" is external or from internal impulses. (**Ref. 1,** p. 252)

18. **(C)** Separation anxiety has its roots in early childhood experiences. Many patterns established during these stages of early attachments are thought to persist in establishing relationships and attachments into adulthood. (**Ref. 1,** pp. 162, 575)

19. **(C)** This classical theory focuses on the gradual moves of the child toward comfortable separation from the parent and an enhanced sense of self. The autistic phase and symbiotic phase precede this rather complex cognitive and affective interaction. (**Ref. 1,** pp. 20–21)

20. **(D)** The child's interest in the world is well established by the point of normal rapproachement. The painful conflict, leading to affective deregulation, is felt to be indicative of the wish to stay with the mother in the face of this interest. (**Ref. 1,** pp. 20–21)

21. **(A)** The anal phase is marked initially by a focus on autoerotic sensations from the anal mucosa (a classical "zone" as described by Freud). From 18 to 36 months, it is a complex mix of internal and external demands, no matter what the parental toilet training style entails. (**Ref. 7,** pp. 131–132)

22. **(A)** "Conscience" is the common equivalent of superego anxiety—anxiety generated when an action the person feels is wrong is done and the expectation is for discovery. The anxiety occurs even without discovery. (**Ref. 7,** p. 137)

23. **(D)** The inability to integrate opposing qualities (eg, "good" and "bad" features of the same person/object), splitting serves a regulatory function for the infant and young child. If it remains a major part of mental activity, pathological adaptations that lack stability are evident (eg, the borderline pathology states). (**Ref. 8,** p. 250)

24. **(B)** Formal thought in the Piagetian framework of development is a hallmark of the adolescent stage; it begins at age 11 and continues through adolescence. The late childhood period would be more consistent with the stages of concrete operations. Freud viewed this period as a relatively quiet phase where sexual drives are channeled into more socially acceptable aims such as sports or school work. (**Ref. 1,** pp. 22–23, 47–48, 159)

25. **(D)** According to the structural theory, the id, ego, and superego are the three provinces of the mind. Ego functions are defined as those personality features that *manage* the instinctual drives arising from the id. This process allows for a buffer between those internal schisms and the reality of the outside world. The superego represents the person's moral conscience. (**Ref. 1,** p. 248)

26. **(C)** The anal stage is felt to relate to ultimate traits around "messy" feelings and activities. It is generally considered to be free of cultural influence, arising out of internal sensations focused on the anal mucosa. (**Ref. 1,** pp. 20–21, 245)

27. **(D)** Kohut's developmental lines focus on the role of narcissism during the movement from infancy to adulthood. His theory is significantly divergent from Freudian theory in regard to the relationships the infant forms, both internally and externally. (**Ref. 1,** p. 257)

28. **(B)** Klein felt that the infant's preverbal development is most critical and is the seat of most pathology. These early object relations are critical and the therapist must interpret these "deep" constructs early in the therapeutic approach—even in children. (**Ref. 1,** pp. 256–257)

29. **(B)** Mahler defines the autistic period as one of comfortable engagement in a unique merging with the caretaker, which is relatively impervious to disruption. Only gradually does the child become aware of a separate existence, when motoric skills heighten. (**Ref. 7,** pp. 20, 130)

30. **(D)** Depression does not require splitting, a feature in the borderline personality organization. This process of separating "all good" from "all bad" is thought to be a normal part of the cogni-

tive process of early infancy. When this process persists into adulthood, it is frequently associated with a borderline personality organization. (**Ref. 1,** p. 545)

31. (C) Sadomasochism is felt to be a regression to the early mixed anal phase sensations of almost painful fullness and the pleasurable discharge phenomena which become eroticized. Also described is oral sadism which is related to the painful pleasure of teething and the experience of discharging frustration through biting. (**Ref. 8,** pp. 170–171)

32. (B) Girls, on average, will reliably precede boys into puberty and early adolescence. This is the stimulus for many typical conflicts of this period, as adolescents turn, with heightened sexual feelings, to "older" peers and away from parents. (**Ref. 1,** p. 51)

33. (E) The study of children placed in foster care can help sort out the genetic/environmental aspects of psychiatric disorder similar to adoption studies. Additionally, study of foster care placement has contributed to the understanding of attachment and separation. (**Ref. 9,** pp. 1996–1997)

34. (D) Children with AIDS often lose their parents, either to death from the infection or to the lifestyle problems (eg, IV drug abuse) that first exposed them to HIV. Placement needs may also include up to 70% of infants who do not develop infection despite their mother's HIV-positive status. (**Ref. 7,** pp. 998–999)

35. (B) Bonding is felt to begin in the immediate postdelivery period. However, the slow growing attachment between an infant and its caretakers occurs with ongoing interaction. Attachment occurs in the face of many obstacles, including sensory deficits, maltreatment, and physical handicaps on both sides. (**Ref. 1,** pp. 43–44)

36. (A) Drives, arising early in Freud's theory, evolved during further study as having sources, objects, aims, and degrees of intensity, depending on their innate and invested cathexis. They are not described in a particular pattern but are often collected under broader headings (eg, aggressive, libidinal, erotic). (**Ref. 1,** p. 242)

37. (C) The typical thinking mode of the unconscious, primary process is felt to be present in normal infant development and is manifest in psychotic states at whatever age or developmental level. It is illogical, ignores external reality, and lacks capacity for delay and/or modulation. (**Ref. 1,** p. 242)

38. (D) Imitative learning takes on personal forms as toddlers adopt, internalize, or reciprocate the activities of their caretakers in the phase of behavioral organization, initiative, and internalization, as described by Stanley Greenspan. They appear to integrate emotional and behavioral opposites, such as love and aggression, during this period. (**Ref. 9,** p. 1699)

39. (B) Attachment requires the infant's emotional investment in the caretaker to be stimulated by the caretaker's emotional investment in the infant (the infant "falls in love" with the caretaker). The caretaker must set aside whatever dependency needs they have for the infant to "care for" them. (**Ref. 9,** p. 1698)

40. (A) In order to achieve homeostasis, infants must regulate the world via their senses. Therefore, babies with sensory deficits must have specialized guidance, as must their parents. (**Ref. 9,** p. 1698)

41. (E) Along with the surge of language development, the use of play enlarges representational capacity and establishes the child's sense of self in the late toddler years. Greenspan sees the role of the caregiver as being supportive of age-appropriate experiences and interpersonal development in this stage. (**Ref. 9,** p. 1699)

42. (B) Pathologically shallow and impersonal involvement with caretakers, coupled with a lack of affective engagement, are signs of failure of attachment in children with autistic disorder as defined by DSM–IV. However, definitive diagnosis is rarely made at this early age. (**Ref. 4,** pp. 66–71)

43. (A) Microcephaly is associated with fetal alcohol syndrome (FAS), along with other facial features. These include short palpebral fissures and midfacial hypoplasia. (**Ref. 9,** p. 1029)

44. (C) Mental retardation is seen in both disorders, as it is in many others prenatally influenced syndromes. These makes a thorough history of the pregnancy critical when evaluating a child with developmental delays. (**Ref. 9,** p. 1029)

45. (C) Short stature also is seen in association with both disorders. This is often a key diagnostic clue. (**Ref. 9,** p. 1742)

46. (D) Neither of these syndromes is transmitted "genetically," in the classical sense of the word. They are felt to represent an effect of the "toxic" intrauterine environment. (**Ref. 9,** p. 1742)

47. (B) Amnesia can have either etiology. The screen memory is a defensive mechanism. (**Ref. 8,** p. 307)

48. (C) Screen memories may pre- or postdate the traumatic event they mask. They often are vivid and compelling, more so than expected for their content, a clue to their real character. Similarly, amnesia can be anterograde (from the event onward in time) or retrograde (from the event backwards). This is felt to be a clue to the etiology in some theoretical systems of understanding. (**Ref. 8,** p. 308)

49. (D) The family romance is a common feature in child development. It is a fantasy that the child is actually of other, usually better off (perhaps royal or famous!), parentage, simply awaiting rescue from the current (dull!) group. (**Ref. 8,** pp. 7, 74, 173)

50. (C) If amnesia is psychogenic, it may yield to psychoanalytic therapy. The screen memory is a common feature in many analyses. (**Ref. 8,** p. 308)

51. (A) Affects are the relatively fleeting and changeable feeling states that clinicians can judge by observation. It is important to observe the quality, quantity, and congruence with physical expression. (**Ref. 1,** p. 300)

52. (C) Both mood and affect are subjectively experienced. More importantly, they should be inquired about to judge their internal congruence with other expressed symptoms. (**Ref. 1,** pp. 300, 303)

53. **(B)** The critical feature in diagnosing mood disorders is the relative stability of the emotional tone in the face of day-to-day supports and stresses. Descriptors include dysphoric, euthymic, expansive, irritable, and others. (**Ref. 1,** p. 303)

54. **(B)** Night terrors are a parasomnia associated with ascendance from stage IV sleep. They are often associated with other parasomnias (eg, sleep walking, sleep talking). (**Ref. 1,** pp. 711–712)

55. **(B)** Night terrors are not remembered. This is in contrast to anxiety dreams, which are useful in that they may contain clues to anxiety features in unconscious mental life. (**Ref. 1,** pp. 711–712)

56. **(C)** Both night terrors and anxiety dreams occur in childhood. Night terrors are most common in children; some consider them a sign of CNS immaturity. Anxiety dreams, also called nightmares, occur at all developmental levels where reliable reports can be obtained based on language skills. (**Ref. 1,** pp. 711–712)

57. **(D)** Neither anxiety dreams nor night terrors is regularly associated with psychopathology, although the person and family may benefit from supportive and educational counseling. If the dream material is disturbing, Freud's theory suggests a failure in the protective function of the dreamwork mechanism. (**Ref. 1,** pp. 241–242, 711–712)

58. **(B)** The early phase is concerned greatly with physiologic changes. By the arrival of mid-adolescence, the teen becomes more interested in new cognitive abilities in abstract thinking and in special relationships. (**Ref. 9,** p. 1711)

59. **(C)** For the late adolescent, abstract thinking is no longer just a "plaything" to juggle social causes with, but a useful tool for problem solving. They also begin to use abstract thinking to project themselves into the future and consider marriage, family, and a profession. (**Ref. 9,** p. 1712)

60. **(A)** Rebellious behavior is a hallmark of early adolescence. It may appear that they are trying to give up their childhood dependence on their parents in one tumultuous step. (**Ref. 9,** p. 1713)

61. (A) Unless the early adolescent has superego supports well in place with effective defenses, his behavior and affect will flounder in the face of pubertal hormonal surges. Prominent coping behaviors include cognitive planning, role rehearsal, humor, and limited self-observation. (**Ref. 9,** p. 1713)

62. (C) Erikson describes expansion of concerns beyond egotistical focus as a major task for those over 60 years old. This perspective is important in Erikson's stage of integrity versus despair and isolation. (**Ref. 1,** p. 68)

63. (A) Establishment of a firm sense of social/sexual self is a major task for people in their twenties and thirties. Erikson saw the focus as the ability to form warm friendships and associations. Jung focused on the task as individuation or seeing oneself as both apart from and a part of society at large. (**Ref. 1,** pp. 56–57)

64. (B) Generativity is a major Eriksonian issue for the 40- to 60-year-old. Erikson defined generativity as the process by which one guides the oncoming generation or improves society. He contrasts this with stagnation. (**Ref. 1,** pp. 60–61)

65. (C) The late adult requires no further posturing to manage life tasks. This increasing autonomy may result from the increased control of the ego and the id. (**Ref. 1,** pp. 68–70)

66. (E) The id, ego, and superego are theoretical constructs. The structured hypothesis does not imply that these constructs actually occupy physical space. (**Ref. 1,** pp. 247–248)

67. (D) The economic hypothesis postulates the development of psychological energy within the mental apparatus. The amount of energy involved speaks to the intensity of the conflict. (**Ref. 8,** p. 120)

68. (A) The dynamic hypothesis describes the interactions between the forces that demand gratification (drives) and those that shape their expression (defenses). Each force is thought of as having an origin, magnitude, and object. (**Ref. 1,** pp. 249–251)

69. (C) The concept of the three systems was Freud's first published model; the existence of the unconscious was a topic of significant debate and controversy. This resulted in Freud's postulation of the structural theory in 1923. (**Ref. 1,** pp. 241–242)

70. (B) Both classical psychosexual development and Erikson's theory note shame as a component of the child's psychology during the anal period. Erikson contrasts this to the child's desire for autonomy between the ages of 1 to 3. (**Ref. 1,** p. 45)

71. (D) Although recent studies cast doubt on this theoretical position, it has appeal to parents and society. It "defines" the classical latency period. (**Ref. 1,** pp. 22–23)

72. (C) Still controversial—with Kohut's theory and others casting doubts on its existence—the oedipal complex, during the genital period of psychosexual development, has strong support in child-based observations, as well as via analytic therapy. (**Ref. 1,** pp. 22–23)

73. (A) The oral stage is posited on observations of the infant as dependent. This model has been challenged by recent demonstrations of surprising infant skills. (**Ref. 1,** p. 20)

74. (C) The boy, threatened by the fear of castration, moves out of the genital period via resolution of the oedipal complex. The formation of the superego and a prevalent identification with the parent of the same sex is the usual outcome of this resolution. (**Ref. 8,** p. 156)

75. (C) Denial is protective during the early phases of grief in the face of overpowering loss. It need not be "broken through," as normally it will resolve. (**Ref. 1,** p. 250)

76. (D) By rationalizing, the drive can be fulfilled with lessened anxiety about the conflict. Rationalization differs from intellectualization, a form of isolation of affect in which objectionable thoughts are permitted conscious awareness, albeit without emotional impact. (**Ref. 1,** p. 251)

77. **(E)** The child gains strength in the face of anxiety and stress by identifying with the father's competence. The boy is able to see himself as more competent (the internalization is central to the individual's basic identity or ego core). (**Ref. 8,** p. 103)

78. **(A)** Undoing is a defense where an attempt is made to "remove" the offensive act. In this case, undoing may serve multiple needs: management of the guilty anxiety about the transgressions, engagement of social support, and a sense of well-being and pride. (**Ref. 8,** p. 49)

79. **(C)** Repression is the banishing from consciousness of impulses that are too anxiety provoking. Repression was felt by Freud to be the prime defense against memories of childhood incest. (**Ref. 1,** p. 251)

80. **(E)** While rationalization is not specific to any mechanism of defense, this process strongly supports repression. This allows the conscious explanation not to be questioned. (**Ref. 1,** p. 251)

81. **(A)** A primitive defense, denial completely avoids awareness of the painful aspect of the reality. Explicit or implicit denial is an integral aspect of all defense mechanism. (**Ref. 8,** p. 50)

82. **(B)** Projection is a characteristic and useful developmental process in children. It is the core of the paranoid patient's pathology. (**Ref. 1,** p. 250)

83. **(D)** Through such displacement, less consequential outcomes are expected. An unconscious decision is made to get angry in a "safe" environment relative to the prospect of potentially losing his/her job. (**Ref. 1,** p. 251)

84. **(A)** Gratification is sustained in the subliminated arena, perhaps not totally but with less risk. Sublimation is considered to be a mature defense. (**Ref. 1,** p. 252)

85. **(E)** A primary defense in the psychoanalytic understanding of the obsessive–compulsive disorder, reaction formation allows settling of anxiety, usually at a cost. Reaction formation is described as a neurotic defense. (**Ref. 1,** p. 251)

86. **(B)** Conversion is a process by which anxiety-provoking mental content is transmuted into physical phenomenon. Conversion symptoms may contain a clue to the stressor/anxiety (eg, blindness when exposed to "unseeable" sexual or aggressive actions). (**Ref. 8,** pp. 46–47, 697)

87. **(C)** Introjection is a normal part of development (eg, a child taking in the parents demands as their own, whether the parents are present or not). Introjection is commonly distorted in children with pathology as "identification with the aggressor," as described by Anna Freud. (**Ref. 8,** p. 102)

88. **(D)** A most dramatic and drastic mental mechanism, dissociation occurs in a variety of "altered states" of consciousness. Most dramatic are those associated with the multiple personality disorder, a controversial diagnosis. (**Ref. 1,** p. 250)

89. **(C)** The oedipal victor fantasy is shared by children of both sexes. Loss of either parent, through death or divorce, can significantly distort development by fulfilling the fantasied wish. (**Ref. 8,** p. 135)

90. **(A)** The family romance fantasy is a cross-culturally identified wish in middle childhood. It is not considered pathological in either sex. (**Ref. 8,** p. 74)

91. **(B)** It is difficult to know if the primal scene report is a fantasy fueled by sound cues and children's shared stories or a true observational experience. In most cultures, children share the parental bed or room, so as to make observation, and possible distortion with aggressive overtones, of parental intercourse common. (**Ref. 7,** p. 135)

92. **(C)** The rapprochement subphase of Mahler's separation–individual schema is marked by volatile mood and attempts to coerce the mother into a controlled position, while being distressed if she allows it. This is a difficult time for many families. (**Ref. 1,** pp. 20–21)

93. **(B)** While in the practicing subphase (10 to 15 months), the mother and toddler can share the new-found delight in mobility

and exploration. The mother is needed in this phase for "emotional refueling," as evidenced by frequent physical contacts around the presentation of toys. (**Ref. 1,** pp. 20–21)

94. **(D)** At the turn into the third year (approximately 24 months), the child's memory stability is such that even small cues, and soon only internal ones, sustain the comfort of the mother's support despite her physical unavailability. Since no memory can fully substitute for the real love object, this phase is an open-ended, lifelong process that may never be fully completed. (**Ref. 1,** pp. 20–21)

95. **(A)** Erikson postulates that problems in the basic ability to trust derive during the stage that Freud described as focusing on the oral zone. This occurs in the first year of life. (**Ref. 1,** p. 20)

96. **(B)** During the anal stage that Freud described, Erikson defined that self-doubt and shame oscillates with a sense of autonomy and pride. A significant example may be the pride associated with mastery of toileting and the self-doubt and shame that are associated with accidents. (**Ref. 1,** pp. 20–21)

97. **(D)** During the period of ages 3 to 5 years, which Freud called the phallic–oedipal stage, Erikson saw the potential for problems with self-directed initiative developing in the face of parental or sibling criticism. Erikson defined his corresponding stage as initiative versus guilt. (**Ref. 1,** p. 22)

98. **(C)** The genital zone takes the lead for both sexes in a move that Erikson sees towards *purpose,* a virtue which can be impaired by an overpunitive conscience. Erikson also notes a strong desire to mimic the adult world that contributes the oedipal struggle. (**Ref. 1,** p. 22)

99. **(B)** The anal zone (and its functioning during toilet training) is critically involved in the development of *will,* which leads to a sense of autonomy. Neurologic and muscular maturation is an important precursor in readiness for this stage. (**Ref. 1,** pp. 20–21)

100. **(D)** For Erikson, the phase of industry versus inferiority depends on the ability to engage in a period of instruction and learn-

ing; this corresponds best to the "latency" stage in psychosexual development. It is also this ability to engage in instruction and learning that has been important to historically starting school at about this age. (**Ref. 1,** pp. 22–23)

101. **(D)** This rich phase of Erikson's theory deals with the adolescent and young adult ages. A major task is to develop an identity separate from the family of origin. This frequently involves identification with peer groups. (**Ref. 1,** p. 23)

102. **(E)** The Prader–Willi syndrome of obesity, usually with dramatic hyperphagia, hypogonadism, and retardation, is not clearly identified as to its underlying genetic pattern. This is in contrast to the other listed disorders. (**Ref. 1,** p. 1028)

103. **(B)** Down syndrome is the common name of the trisomy 21 chromosomal anomaly. It is the most frequently recognized cause of developmental delays. (**Ref. 1,** p. 1027)

104. **(A)** Short girls with webbed necks and slowed sexual development have the classical Turner syndrome if they lack one X chromosome—the XO pattern. Frequently, medical management is necessary to assist them with their infertility and absence of secondary sexual characteristics. (**Ref. 1,** p. 685)

105. **(D)** Fragile X is the second most common known syndrome causing developmental delay. Increasing evidence shows cognitive effects in both carrier females and their sons/brothers. (**Ref. 1,** pp. 1027–1028)

2

Cultural, Environmental, and Interpersonal Factors

Elizabeth Caspary
Kathryn C. Krieg

DIRECTIONS (Questions 1 through 27) Each of the questions or incomplete statements below is followed by five suggested answers or completions. Select the ONE that is best in each case.

---

1. Faris and Dunham found that
    A. schizophrenia is more prevalent in central city slum areas
    B. bipolar affective disorder is more common in central city slum areas
    C. schizophrenia and bipolar disorder with psychosis are manifestations of the same disorder
    D. schizophrenia is more prevalent in affluent suburban areas
    E. bipolar affective disorder is more prevalent in affluent suburban areas

2. Basic principles of community psychiatry include
   A. services offered are based on the preferences of mental health center staff members
   B. availability of treatment close to where the patient lives
   C. services limited to inpatient hospital and outpatient clinic treatments for mental disorders
   D. minimization of the different roles of various mental health professionals
   E. limited research opportunities

3. In general, immigrant groups
   A. have lower suicide rates than native-born citizens
   B. have a high incidence of borderline personality disorder
   C. show clear differences in genetic predisposition to specific mental disorders
   D. tend to have high rates of psychotic illness at the time of entry into a new country
   E. are less likely to be admitted to a psychiatric hospital than native-born citizens

4. Which of the following was reported by Hollingshead and Redlich?
   A. the prevalence of neurotic disorders is higher in families of the lowest socioeconomic group
   B. mental disorders in lower socioeconomic families generally are treated in outpatient clinics
   C. mental disorders in lower socioeconomic families are characterized by a brief duration of illness
   D. the prevalence of schizophrenia is higher in families of the lowest socioeconomic group
   E. social class and treatment setting of mental disorders are unrelated

5. Which of the following psychiatric disorders have the same prevalence among both men and women?
   A. unipolar depression
   B. bipolar affective disorder
   C. bulimia nervosa
   D. alcohol dependence
   E. phobic disorder

6. The LEAST helpful in dealing with an agitated, threatening patient is
   A. focusing on an underlying feeling state or affect
   B. allowing the patient to verbally ventilate angry feelings
   C. attempting to calm the person through rationalization or intellectualization
   D. offering appropriate food or drink
   E. expression of fear by the staff if the patient has a weapon

7. During adolescence, MOST individuals experience
   A. a high incidence of turmoil and severe crisis
   B. a reactivation of the Oedipus complex
   C. severe character pathology
   D. recapitulation of infantile neurosis
   E. stable, consistent, and empathic relationships with parents

8. The family unit that is composed of persons of two generations and two genders is known as the
   A. basic family
   B. nuclear family
   C. extended family
   D. common family
   E. primary family

9. Which of the following is true of the homeless?
   A. approximately 5% of the homeless are mentally ill, according to a 1991 study
   B. the homeless mentally ill usually have major depression
   C. homeless mentally ill prefer their independence on the streets
   D. there is a very high rate of alcoholism and alcohol-related medical illnesses among the homeless mentally ill
   E. all of the above

10. From the studies of sociobiology we have learned
    A. a great deal about animal behavior but little that applies to human society
    B. that evolutionary concepts apply to most mammals, but not to human beings
    C. that Darwin's concept of natural selection was in error
    D. that behavior derives from interactions between an organism's genotype and its environment
    E. that individuals consciously choose behavior patterns that will result in greater evolutionary success

11. Which of the following is an example of primary prevention of mental disorders?
    A. methadone clinic
    B. day hospital
    C. nursing home placement
    D. Head Start program
    E. child guidance clinic

12. Secondary prevention of mental disorders is defined as
    A. those efforts which prevent the onset of a mental disorder
    B. those efforts which strengthen an individual's capacity to withstand or cope with stress
    C. early identification and prompt treatment of a disorder
    D. reduction of residual defects or disabilities due to a disorder
    E. prevention of the transmission of mental disorders

13. All the following have been factors preventing adequate treatment of the chronically, severely mentally ill EXCEPT
    A. deinstitutionalization
    B. inadequate housing
    C. discharging mentally ill to shelters
    D. treatment team assessing patients by observation rather than interviewing patient
    E. having no mailbox

14. Cognitive changes found in the elderly include
    A. a decline in perceptual motor skills
    B. a decline in verbal performance
    C. a decline in most intellectual functions
    D. an inability to learn new material
    E. poor recall of past events

15. Which of the following is a major developmental issue in aging?
    A. cessation of sexual activity
    B. development and use of new ego defenses
    C. reminiscing and life review
    D. development of new coping skills
    E. absence of sexual fantasies

16. The MOST consistent symptom that occurs as a result of menopause is
    A. hot flashes
    B. dizzy spells
    C. depression
    D. palpitations
    E. headaches

17. Which of the following statements regarding suicide is TRUE?
    A. Native Americans have a lower suicide rate than white Americans
    B. most suicide victims do not have a known psychiatric disorder
    C. over the last decade, suicide rates have declined for all age groups
    D. physicians have a lower overall suicide rate than the general population
    E. suicide is among the top ten causes of death in the United States

18. Which of the following statements regarding postpartum psychiatric disorders is TRUE?
    A. patients with a known history of schizophrenia who have experienced a postpartum psychiatric illness are at the highest risk for a recurrence
    B. hormonal changes occurring during the peak presentation of postpartum psychosis include a drop in estrogen and prolactin levels and a rise in progesterone levels
    C. women with borderline personality disorder are more likely to experience postpartum disorders
    D. during the first postpartum month, a women has a higher likelihood of psychiatric hospitalization than at any other time in her life
    E. prepartum depression and anxiety lead to an increased incidence of postpartum disorders

19. Primary prevention in mental health encompasses
    A. screening and early diagnosis
    B. promotion of general well-being and the acquisition of coping skills
    C. early treatment
    D. reduction of residual disabilities
    E. shortening the duration of illness

20. Death from suicide is
    A. not a leading cause of death in the 15-to-24-year-old group
    B. more likely among individuals who have previously attempted suicide
    C. an infrequent cause of death among the elderly
    D. more common in the Middle Atlantic States than in the Western Mountain States
    E. more common in rural areas than in urban areas

21. Which of the following statements about adolescent sexuality is TRUE?
    A. availability of sex education and contraceptives have resulted in a decline in teenage pregnancy
    B. teenagers generally are promiscuous in their relationships
    C. half of teenage marriages will end in divorce within five years

    D. the rate for teenage births in the United States is much lower than that in England, France, or Sweden

    E. pregnant teenagers have less risk of toxemia, premature birth, and perinatal morbidity than more mature women

22. Psychiatric sequelae following an abortion include

    A. depressive symptoms beginning almost immediately

    B. depressive symptoms occurring around the time when the baby would have been born

    C. none for the male partners

    D. depressive symptoms during subsequent pregnancies

    E. brief psychotic reactions after the procedure

23. Which of the following pairs of coping defenses and mechanisms is MOST correlated with good adjustment in adulthood?

    A. denial, suppression

    B. projection, altruism

    C. dissociation, humor

    D. intellectualization, depression

    E. suppression, altruism

24. Which of the following is TRUE of families in the United States today?

    A. ten percent of children in the United States live with just one parent

    B. of the children in single-parent homes, 60% live with their mothers and 40% live with their fathers

    C. about half of all children in the United States will live in a single-parent household by the time they reach adulthood

    D. twenty percent of all marriages end in divorce

    E. most families today are patriarchal primary families

25. Family homeostasis refers to

    A. understanding individuals as part of a family matrix

    B. understanding symptoms in terms of the family as a whole

    C. transference between family members

    D. mechanisms that maintain the equilibrium of the family

    E. countertransference between the therapist and family members

26. Which of the following is a characteristic of an abnormal grief reaction?
   A. hypochondriacal complaints resembling symptoms of the last illness of the deceased
   B. preoccupation with the image of the deceased
   C. increased emotional distance from others
   D. somatic distress
   E. symptoms persisting beyond six weeks

27. Which of the following statements is TRUE regarding psychiatric disorders in the elderly?
   A. among the elderly between ages 90 and 95, 80% have a diagnosis of dementia
   B. among elderly patients with dementia, 75% suffer from Alzheimer's disease
   C. the elderly tend to use more lethal methods in their suicide attempts than younger individuals
   D. the prognosis for elderly patients with diagnosed depression is better than that for younger patients
   E. episodes of mania no longer occur once an individual reaches the sixth or seventh decade

---

DIRECTIONS (Questions 28 through 32): For each numbered clinical vignette, select the lettered psychiatric sign or symptom which is most accurately described. Each lettered heading may be selected once, more than once, or not at all.

   A. clang association
   B. delusion
   C. hallucination
   D. ideas of reference
   E. illusion

28. A 21-year-old man sees a U.S. Army poster which says "Uncle Sam Wants You." He believes this contains a special message just for him

29. A 19-year-old woman hears the voice of God telling her to refuse to take psychotropic medications

30. A 35-year-old psychotic woman answers an interview question with the following statement: "It was a Nabisco-Disco-Crisco"

31. A 76-year-old woman suffers from psoriasis. She misperceives the skin symptoms as a sign that spiders have invaded her skin

32. A 40-year-old woman believes that she suffers from carpal tunnel syndrome despite objective medical evidence to the contrary.

DIRECTIONS (Questions 33 through 36): Each lettered term comes from studies of grief and the mourning process. Match each numbered definition with the term with which it is most closely associated. Each lettered heading may be selected once, more than once, or not at all.

    A. normal grief
    B. abnormal grief
    C. anticipatory grief
    D. sudden crisis
    E. situational crisis

33. Postponement of the experience of grief or absence of grief

34. Reaction experienced in the face of an impending loss

35. Stress experienced by a number of persons in a population when exposed to a precipitous change in social context caused by a disaster or a major social or economic change

36. Somatic distress, marked by sighing respiration, exhaustion, and various digestive symptoms

---

DIRECTIONS (Questions 37 through 51): Match the following as to risk for suicide.

    A. high risk
    B. low risk

37. Male

38. Married

39. Unemployed

40. Living alone

41. Family history of suicide

42. Chronic medical illness

43. Hopelessness

44. Alcoholism

45. Depressive disorder

46. Catholic

47. Wrist cutting

48. Firearms

49. Impulsive

50. Imminent rescue

51. Multiple previous attempts

Cultural, Environmental, and Interpersonal Factors

Explanatory Answers

1. (A) In their study *Mental Disorders in Urban Areas,* Faris and Dunham reported that there are fewer people with schizophrenia toward the outskirts of the city; no definite pattern was noted for bipolar disorders. (**Ref. 1,** pp. 193, 207)

2. (B) Community psychiatry principles include: responsibility to a population of a given geographic area, comprehensive services (eg, inpatient, outpatient, emergency, partial hospitalization, and education), multidisciplinary team approach, objective program evaluation and research, and treatment available close to patients' homes. (**Ref. 1,** pp. 202–203)

3. (D) Overall suicide rates among immigrants are significantly higher than those of native-born citizens. Some studies have shown that immigrants are more likely to be antisocial than natives. Immigrant groups tend to have high rates of psychotic illness at the time of entry to a new country; over time rates approximate those of native-born citizens. (**Ref. 9,** pp. 15:9, 19:3, 20:7–9)

4. (D) Hollingshead and Redlich found a strong association between higher social class, less severe disorders, and private office treatment settings. There was also a strong association between lower social class, more severe disorders, longer duration of disorders, and long hospital stays in public institutions. (**Ref. 1,** pp. 193–194; **Ref. 9,** p. 319)

5. **(B)** Unipolar depression, eating disorders, and anxiety disorders have a higher prevalence among women. Alcohol abuse/dependence has a higher prevalence among men. The ratio of females to males is equal for bipolar disorder. (**Ref. 5,** pp. 322, 437, 769–774)

6. **(C)** Trying to calm an agitated, threatening person by rationalization or intellectualization may increase their sense of not being understood. Focusing on underlying affect and allowing expression of angry affect will help dissipate hostile feelings. Offering food or drink that could not be used as a weapon (eg, mug of hot coffee) may give the patient a sense of being cared for. Appealing to the patient's sense of fairness may allow him to more easily give up the weapon. (**Ref. 3,** pp. 555–556)

7. **(E)** Daniel and Judith Offer's study of adolescents revealed that the incidence of turmoil and severe crisis is quite low. They observed that the overwhelming majority of adolescents are free of dramatic conflicts and have stable relationships with their parents. (**Ref. 5,** pp. 638–640)

8. **(B)** The nuclear family consists of father, mother, and children and is a universal unit in all cultures. (**Ref. 9,** p. 1537)

9. **(D)** In some studies, as high as 45% of the homeless are alcoholic and 33% have alcohol-related medical illnesses. Of the homeless, one study in 1991 showed 33% to be mentally ill. The most common diagnosis is schizophrenia. Severe regression and inability to attend to basic needs are factors in causing homelessness in the population. (**Ref. 1,** pp. 204–205)

10. **(D)** Sociobiology emphasizes an evolutionary basis for understanding behavior of all animals, including humans. The concept of natural selection is central to sociobiology. Natural selection results in certain types of behavior without an awareness of the underlying motivation. (**Ref. 1,** p. 185; **Ref. 9,** pp. 338–339)

11. **(D)** The goal of primary prevention is to prevent the onset of a disease or disorder, and thereby reduce its incidence. (**Ref. 1,** p. 203; **Ref. 9,** pp. 2067–2068)

12. **(C)** Secondary prevention is defined as early identification and prompt treatment of illness or disorder. The goal of tertiary prevention is to reduce the prevalence of residual defects or disabilities due to illness or disorder. Primary preventive efforts include those that strengthen an individual's capacity to withstand or cope with stress, decrease disease transmission, and prevent the onset of a disease or disorder. (**Ref. 1,** p. 203; **Ref. 9,** pp. 2067–2070)

13. **(D)** Because of problems with verbal communication with the mentally ill, assessment by observation may be essential to treating the patient. This population will also require assistance with meeting basic needs, such as obtaining appropriate housing, and finding a means to obtain minimal financial support (eg, a mailbox to send checks to). (**Ref. 1,** pp. 203–205)

14. **(A)** Intellectual functions show little or no decline in individuals over age 60, although perceptual motor skills may decline. Learning can occur even at advanced ages, provided strategies are followed which facilitate learning in the elderly. The elderly have difficulty with short-term memory, but recall of past events is quite good. (**Ref. 5,** p. 667)

15. **(C)** Sexual behavior in the elderly corresponds to their individual sex life when they were younger. Coping skills and ego defensive mechanisms are established very early and persist throughout life. (**Ref. 5,** pp. 667–669)

16. **(A)** Hot flashes is the most consistent symptom associated with menopause, occurring in about 75% of women in our culture. The other symptoms listed are not related to menopause. (**Ref. 1,** p. 61; **Ref. 9,** p. 1337)

17. **(E)** Native Americans have a higher suicide rate than white Americans of all age groups. An overwhelming majority of suicide victims suffer from a concomitant psychiatric illness. Suicide rates have been relatively stable over the last decade, except for an increase in adolescent victims. Physicians have a higher-than-

normal rate of suicide. Suicide is the ninth leading cause of death in the United States. (**Ref. 1,** pp. 803–805)

18. **(D)** Patients with a known history of bipolar illness who have experienced a postpartum psychiatric illness are at the highest risk for a recurrence. A dramatic drop in estrogen and progesterone levels and a large increase in prolactin occurs during the peak presentation of postpartum psychosis. Women with obsessive–compulsive traits are more likely to experience postpartum disorders. Findings about whether prepartum depression or anxiety leads to an increase in postpartum disorders are inconsistent. (**Ref. 1,** pp. 494–496; **Ref. 9,** pp. 852–855)

19. **(B)** Early diagnosis and treatment and shortening the duration of illness constitute secondary prevention. Reduction of residual disability constitutes tertiary prevention. (**Ref. 1,** p. 203; **Ref. 9,** pp. 2067–2069)

20. **(B)** Suicide is the third leading cause of death during the age period 15 to 24 years. Suicide rates are the highest in the over-65 age group. The western mountain states have suicide rates much higher than the middle Atlantic states. The rural population has a lower suicide rate than the urban population. (**Ref. 1,** pp. 803– 806)

21. **(C)** The rate of births for teenagers in the United States has increased dramatically over the last two decades, and greatly surpasses the rate in England, France, or Sweden. This has occurred despite widespread availability of sex education and contraceptives. Toxemia, premature birth, and perinatal morbidity are more frequent in adolescents. (**Ref. 2,** p. 1337; **Ref. 5,** pp. 649–651)

22. **(B)** Moderate depression may be seen around the time that the baby would have been born. Symptoms are more severe in the case of a forced abortion or a second trimester abortion. Abortion is not a neutral event for male partners. (**Ref. 1,** pp. 30–33; **Ref. 9,** pp. 1337–1338)

23. **(E)** In a 30-year prospective study of healthy American men, Vaillant found that suppression and altruism were more mature coping mechanisms. Humor and sublimation also belonged in this group. (**Ref. 5,** pp. 202–203)

24. **(C)** About a quarter of the children in the United States live with just one parent. Of children in single-parent homes, nearly 90% live with their mothers, while close to 10% live with their fathers. One out of every two marriages ends in divorce. A male's position as unchallenged authority in the household (patriarchal primary) has decreased. (**Ref. 1,** pp. 58–60; **Ref. 9,** pp. 1409–1412)

25. **(D)** From a systems approach, the family works to preserve an equilibrium. Any disturbance in the balance of forces activates counterforces which reduce the disequilibrium and bring the system back into balance. (**Ref. 5,** pp. 475–477)

26. **(A)** Items B through E can be seen in a normal grief reaction. Hypochondriacal complaints are felt to be part of a distorted or pathologic grief reaction. (**Ref. 3,** pp. 595–598)

27. **(C)** Among the elderly between the ages 90 and 95, about 39% have a diagnosable dementia. Among the elderly who suffer from dementia, about 57% suffer from Alzheimer's disease. There tends to be an increased lethality in the methods used in suicide attempts by the elderly. The prognosis for elderly patients diagnosed with depression is not as favorable as that for younger individuals. Manic episodes in the sixth or seventh decade of life are not unusual. (**Ref. 3,** pp. 342–345)

28. **(D), 29. (C), 30. (A), 31. (E), 32. (B)** Clang associations are rhyming or punning associations of one word with another, with no logical connection. A delusion is a false belief held firmly despite contradictory evidence. A hallucination is a false sensory perception of what is not there. Ideas of reference are beliefs that external events have personal significance. An illusion is a perceptual distortion of something that is there. (**Ref. 2,** pp. 477–479)

33. **(B), 34. (C), 35. (E), 36. (A)** Anticipatory grief and situational crisis are terms that come from Lindemann's classic study of the survivors of the Coconut Grove fire in 1944. Current DSM–IV nosology subsumes some of situational crisis under posttraumatic stress disorder. Somatic symptoms such as insomnia, anorexia, weight loss, fatigue, and gastrointestinal symptoms

can accompany normal grief. Abnormal grief reactions can occur when the feelings of grief are too overwhelming and are, therefore, repressed and postponed. (**Ref. 3,** pp. 595–598, **Ref. 5,** pp. 751, 757, 787)

37. (A),   38. (B),   39. (A),   40. (A),   41. (A),   42. (A), 43. (A),   44. (A),   45. (A),   46. (B),   47. (B),   48. (A), 49. (A),   50. (B),   51. (A) Risk factors can only be guidelines to helping assess the suicidality of any individual. A patient who has made a suicide attempt should never be discharged from an emergency room without a thorough psychiatric evaluation. The lethality of the method of attempt is one of the most important considerations. For example, the purchase or use of a gun is a serious indicator. The patient's perception of lethality is also a factor. An individual may overdose on a benzodiazepine in the belief that a prescription drug is automatically lethal. Another may overdose with aspirin in a suicidal gesture only to die from medical complications. The imminence of possible rescue is another important consideration. A person who overdoses in a hotel room usually has a more serious intent than someone who overdoses with a significant other in an adjoining room. In epidemiological studies, gender, unemployment, family suicide history, chronic mental illness, hopelessness, alcoholism, depression, impulsivity, and multiple previous attempts have all been shown to increase the risk of suicide. Male risk of suicide exceeds that of females. Those who are single, widowed, separated, or divorced have higher risk than those who are married. Catholics have a low suicide risk compared to other religious backgrounds. (**Ref. 3,** p. 563)

3

Diagnosis and Evaluation
Joseph B. Layde
Gunnar Larson

DIRECTIONS (Questions 1 through 51): Each of the questions or incomplete statements below is followed by five suggested answers or completions. Select the ONE that is best in each case.

---

1. Mrs. Jones has come to your office many times for a variety of complaints. In spite of multiple examinations and laboratory tests, you have not been able to find an organic basis for any of her symptoms. She responds to your favorable report of her tests with a new barrage of symptoms. At this point, it would be MOST useful to say

   A. "Mrs. Jones, there is absolutely nothing wrong with you"
   B. "I think you should see a psychiatrist"
   C. "I have another medicine I would like you to try"
   D. "I'm puzzled, Mrs. Jones, about your response to the good news. Do you have any ideas about that?"
   E. "I think your problem is emotional, Mrs. Jones. I can't find anything wrong with you"

2. The mental status examination includes all of the following EX-
   CEPT
   A. general appearance, manner, and attitude
   B. affect, thought processes
   C. memory
   D. judgment, insight
   E. personal history

3. The summary of a patient's problems, important influences, psy-
   chodynamics, diagnostic classification, expected transference re-
   lationships, and prognosis constitute
   A. the mental status examination
   B. the psychiatric history
   C. the psychosocial formulation
   D. the psychiatric examination
   E. none of the above

4. All of the following statements concerning the Wechsler Adult
   Intelligence Scale–Revised (WAIS-R) are true EXCEPT
   A. the verbal scale includes items that require a response in
      words
   B. the performance scale includes items that require a nonver-
      bal response
   C. the performance scale includes tests consisting of arranging
      pictures in a meaningful sequence and assembling parts of a
      puzzle
   D. the verbal scale includes arithmetic, similarities, and repro-
      ducing designs with blocks
   E. the subtest scores provide an opportunity to screen for or-
      ganic deficits

5. The WAIS-R
   A. tests only innate intellectual ability
   B. includes only verbal tests
   C. is of little value in differentiating types of psychopathology
   D. is a projective test
   E. is none of the above

6. In the thematic apperception test (TAT), the patient
   A. detects the pattern in a series of numbers
   B. interrupts a story when he can guess the ending
   C. draws a picture to illustrate a story
   D. constructs a story to accompany a picture
   E. does none of the above

7. Which of the following techniques is MOST useful in differentiating functional from organic impotence?
   A. Minnesota Multiphasic Personality Inventory–2 (MMPI–2)
   B. Rorschach
   C. nocturnal penile tumescence recording
   D. Bender gestalt
   E. skull x-rays

8. Which of the following is NOT a test for assessing brain damage?
   A. Bender gestalt
   B. Halstead–Reitan
   C. Luria–Nebraska
   D. trail-making test
   E. Rorschach

9. Which of the following is NOT a sign of starvation found in some patients with anorexia nervosa?
   A. hypothermia
   B. dependent edema
   C. bradycardia
   D. lanugo hair
   E. hypertension

10. Sedative–hypnotic intoxication induces each of the following signs EXCEPT
    A. slurred speech
    B. extreme wakefulness
    C. incoordination
    D. unsteady gait
    E. impairment in attention or memory

11. The illegal drug called "ice" is a smokeable form of
    A. cocaine
    B. methamphetamine
    C. heroin
    D. diazepam
    E. warfarin

12. All of the following are self-help groups important in the comprehensive treatment of drug abuse EXCEPT
    A. Alcoholics Anonymous
    B. Overeaters Anonymous
    C. Cocaine Anonymous
    D. Narcotics Anonymous
    E. Drugs Anonymous

13. Which of the following is MOST useful in measuring cerebral blood flow?
    A. CT scan
    B. MRI
    C. SPECT
    D. skull films
    E. physical examination

14. Which of the following is NOT an abnormal motor behavior seen in mental illness?
    A. catalepsy
    B. waxy flexibility
    C. automatism
    D. reaction formation
    E. stereotypy

15. Which of the following is characteristic of the dexamethasone suppression test for depression?
    A. high specificity
    B. a positive or abnormal response if a patient has a reduction in serum cortisol levels after receiving oral dexamethasone
    C. frequent false-positive results
    D. rare false-negative results
    E. high sensitivity

16. Which of the following is NOT a frequently used diagnostic study in the workup of individuals with abnormal mental states?
  A. liver function tests
  B. serum vitamin B_{12}
  C. serum folate level
  D. bronchoscopy
  E. chest x-ray

17. Which of the following is NOT a frequently found sign in patients with bulimia?
  A. sores on the hand
  B. weight fluctuations
  C. swelling of salivary glands
  D. absence of a patellar reflex
  E. erosion of tooth enamel

18. Which of the following is associated with a particularly poor prognosis of schizophrenia?
  A. acute onset
  B. affective symptoms
  C. clouded sensorium
  D. positive family history of schizophrenia
  E. marriage

19. All of the following conditions mimic schizophrenia EXCEPT
  A. amphetamine intoxication
  B. steroid-induced mental changes
  C. temporal lobe epilepsy
  D. L-dopa treatment-related mental changes
  E. heroin intoxication

20. Patients with a major depression usually present with a history of each of the following EXCEPT
  A. insomnia
  B. tearfulness
  C. suicidal thoughts
  D. visual hallucinations
  E. fatigue

21. In evaluating a patient with a sexual dysfunction, which of the following approaches should be taken?
    A. ask intimate questions about the patient's sexual history without shame
    B. avoid questions about homosexuality
    C. accept the patient's attitudes about sex, even when he/she is dysfunctional
    D. apologize after asking delicate sexual questions
    E. avoid questions about painful intercourse

22. Which of the following statements is NOT true about homosexuality?
    A. it is considered a mental disorder by the American Psychiatric Association
    B. it is a risk factor for AIDS
    C. it is distinct from transsexualism
    D. it is a risk factor for genital herpes infection
    E. ego-dystonic homosexuality is classified in DSM-IV as a sexual disorder not otherwise specified

23. What proportion of schizophrenic patients eventually commit suicide?
    A. about 1%
    B. about 3%
    C. about 5%
    D. about 10%
    E. about 50%

24. Which of the following is NOT a recognized subtype of schizophrenia?
    A. paranoid
    B. disorganized
    C. catatonic
    D. phlegmatic
    E. undifferentiated

25. Which of the following is a positive symptom of schizophrenia?
    A. flattened affect
    B. poverty of speech
    C. apathy

D. impaired hygiene

E. auditory hallucinations

26. Which of the following is characteristic of positron emission to-
    mography (PET) scans?

    A. radiation exposure

    B. three-hour imaging time

    C. low cost

    D. inability to locate sites of metabolism

    E. wide availability

27. Which of the following patients would be a more appropriate can-
    didate for a computed tomography (CT) scan than for magnetic
    resonance imaging (MRI)?

    A. a young woman with multiple sclerosis

    B. a child with a suspected abnormality in the size of his ventri-
    cles

    C. a man with an implanted cardiac pacemaker

    D. a woman with suspected temporal lobe disease

    E. a child with autism

28. Which of the following is a sign of AIDS dementia on a single
    photon emission computed tomography (SPECT) scan?

    A. generalized decreased cerebral perfusion

    B. generalized increased cerebral perfusion

    C. decreased frontal perfusion

    D. patchy areas of decreased perfusion

    E. generalized cortical atrophy

29. Compared to suicide attempters, suicide completers are more likely
    to be

    A. younger

    B. male

    C. impulsive in planning the attempt

    D. likely to act when help is available

    E. suffering from a personality disorder

30. Compared to the general population, the suicide rate in patients with AIDS is
    A. about one-half as high
    B. about as high
    C. nearly ten times as high
    D. nearly 20 times as high
    E. nearly 60 times as high

31. Which of the following is NOT characteristic of phencyclidine (PCP)?
    A. it is an analogue of the anesthetic ketamine
    B. it is frequently smoked
    C. its abuse may cause a toxic psychosis
    D. hypertension is rarely seen in patients with PCP intoxication
    E. coma is sometimes seen in PCP toxicity

32. Which of the following is NOT true of the Bender gestalt test?
    A. it consists of a series of nine geometric patterns
    B. the patient copies patterns from models
    C. most people have difficulty drawing the figures
    D. rotations of figures may suggest perceptual difficulties
    E. gross distortions of copied figures may suggest perceptual or motor problems

33. Which of the following is NOT likely to be useful in the management of demented patients?
    A. low-stimulus situations
    B. consistency of routine
    C. treatment of accompanying depression
    D. treatment of accompanying psychosis
    E. anticholinergic medication

34. Which of the following characterizes the genetic transmission of Huntington's disease?
    A. X-linked recessive transmission
    B. X-linked dominant transmission
    C. autosomal recessive transmission
    D. autosomal dominant transmission
    E. none of the above

35. What is the IQ cutoff point used to define mental retardation?
  A. below 60
  B. below 65
  C. below 70
  D. below 75
  E. below 80

36. MOST depressed patients studied in sleep laboratories show
  A. increased time of sleep before the first REM period
  B. decreased time of sleep until the first REM period
  C. no REM sleep
  D. no non-REM sleep
  E. none of the above

37. What percentage of women in "normal couples" report inability to have orgasms?
  A. about 15%
  B. about 30%
  C. nearly 50%
  D. 75%
  E. 90%

38. What percentage of men in "normal couples" report that they ejaculate too quickly?
  A. about 10%
  B. about 20%
  C. about 30%
  D. more than 35%
  E. more than 50%

39. Involuntary muscle contractions of the outer third of the vagina sufficient to prevent penile insertion constitute a condition known as
  A. vaginismus
  B. dyspareunia
  C. anhedonia
  D. frigidity
  E. anorgasmia

40. What percentage of children are mentally retarded?
   A. about 1%
   B. about 2%
   C. about 3%
   D. about 4%
   E. about 5%

41. What percentage of mentally retarded individuals suffer from mild mental retardation (IQs from 50 to 69)?
   A. 20%
   B. 40%
   C. 60%
   D. 80%
   E. almost 100%

42. A 49-year-old white man presents with detailed complaints of difficulty thinking, which have been of short duration. He reports memory gaps, but his attention and concentration are well preserved. He makes little effort to perform simple tasks in the mental status examination. The MOST likely diagnosis is
   A. delirium
   B. dementia
   C. pseudodementia
   D. schizophrenia
   E. mental retardation

43. A 25-year-old Chinese man, who has just arrived in the United States, complains that his penis is retracting into his abdomen and fears this will likely kill him. He mentions that several young men in his Chinese village had the same complaint when he left China. The MOST likely diagnosis is
   A. hysterical koro
   B. antisocial personality disorder
   C. alcohol abuse
   D. amphetamine abuse
   E. schizophrenia

44. Which of the following is NOT a typical sign in a patient with moderate opiate intoxication?
   A. drowsiness
   B. pupillary dilation

C. slurred speech
D. impaired attention
E. impaired memory

45. Intravenous heroin use is likely to produce all of the following subjective symptoms EXCEPT
    A. a feeling of flushing
    B. an orgasmic sensation in the abdomen
    C. euphoria
    D. intense pain in the limbs
    E. a profound sense of well-being

46. Heroin addicts may be detoxified with the aid of pharmacological treatment with
    A. cocaine
    B. clonidine
    C. naloxone
    D. marijuana
    E. PCP

47. Properties of methadone that make it useful in heroin withdrawal include all of the following EXCEPT
    A. its short half-life
    B. its ability to be administered orally once daily
    C. its easy titration
    D. its action as an opiate agonist
    E. its control of the autonomic symptoms of heroin withdrawal

48. Which one of the following psychological tests is a projective test?
    A. Minnesota Multiphasic Personality Inventory–2 (MMPI–2)
    B. Wechsler Adult Intelligence Scale–Revised (WAIS–R)
    C. Rorschach
    D. Halstead–Reitan
    E. Luria–Nebraska

49. Which of the following personality disorders is marked by a pervasively dramatic lifestyle?
   A. paranoid personality disorder
   B. avoidant personality disorder
   C. schizoid personality disorder
   D. histrionic personality disorder
   E. schizotypal personality disorder

50. Which of the following statements is TRUE?
   A. persons with avoidant personality disorder often long for more human contact
   B. persons with schizoid personality disorder often long for more human contact
   C. persons with antisocial personality disorder rarely are involved in difficulties with the law
   D. persons with borderline personality disorder have a pervasively subdued way of relating to others
   E. persons with paranoid personality disorder generally are very trusting

51. Which of the following causes of mental retardation can be prevented by dietary control?
   A. congenital rubella
   B. Tay–Sachs disease
   C. phenylketonuria
   D. trisomy 21
   E. Lesch–Nyhan syndrome

DIRECTIONS (Questions 52 through 54): This section consists of a clinical situation, followed by a series of questions. Study the situation and select the ONE best answer to each question following it.

A 20-year-old man who recently moved to the area came to a general medical clinic complaining of insomnia, lack of appetite, vague muscular aches, lack of zest, and feelings of sadness and loneliness. The examining student made the diagnosis of adjustment disorder with depressed mood and sympathized with the patient for his not yet having made new friends.

Two weeks later, the young man returned, reporting, "I did like you said, and now do *we* have trouble!" He said that he had found a friend, a young girl who was a minor and the local sheriff's daughter. On their first date, they proceeded to have intercourse in the living room of the sheriff's home and to make enough noise to get caught.

52. The examining student would MOST appropriately respond at this time as follows:
   A. "What do you mean *we*?"
   B. "I didn't tell you to do anything"
   C. "You sure goofed up"
   D. "Tell me more about what happened"
   E. "How are we going to get out of this mess?"

53. Which of the following features of this patient is LEAST consistent with the diagnosis of a major depression?
   A. insomnia
   B. lack of appetite
   C. lack of zest
   D. feelings of sadness
   E. sexual appetite

54. Each of the following characteristics can be seen in this patient's presentation EXCEPT
   A. impulsiveness
   B. self-destructive behavior
   C. antisocial behavior
   D. projection
   E. auditory hallucinations

DIRECTIONS (Questions 55 through 59): Each of the questions or incomplete statements below is followed by five suggested answers or completions. Select the ONE that is best in each case.

---

55. Which of the following is TRUE regarding Wilson's disease?
    A. it is a disease of manganese metabolism
    B. it is an autosomal dominant disorder
    C. it causes hepatic dysfunction, dystonia, cerebellar ataxia, intention tremor, and psychiatric symptoms
    D. age of onset generally is between 40 and 50 years
    E. it is an untreatable disorder

56. All of the following are correct statements about hypothyroidism EXCEPT
    A. hypothyroidism may mimic mood disorder
    B. hypothyroidism may present with a psychosis
    C. hypothyroidism may present as hypomania
    D. ten percent of patients with hypothyroidism have residual neuropsychiatric symptoms after hormone replacement therapy
    E. weight loss and a rise in pitch of the voice are typical in hypothyroidism

57. What is the alcohol content of beverages from which alcohol is MOST rapidly absorbed?
    A. 5%
    B. 10%
    C. 15% to 30%
    D. 30% to 50%
    E. 85% to 95%

58. Which of the following is TRUE regarding caffeine withdrawal?
    A. caffeine is a very strong reinforcer
    B. the most characteristic symptoms of caffeine withdrawal are headache and fatigue
    C. caffeine withdrawal syndrome generally lasts less than a day
    D. caffeine tolerance is rare in heavy users of caffeine-containing drinks
    E. ten percent of adult Americans consume more than 500 milligrams of caffeine per day

59. All of the following statements about hyperthyroidism are true EXCEPT
  A. insomnia is seen frequently in patients with hyperthyroidism
  B. energy levels often are subjectively decreased in patients with hyperthyroidism
  C. rapid speech is unusual in patients with hyperthyroidism
  D. overtreatment with thyroid hormone can sometimes mimic endogenous hyperthyroidism
  E. manic excitement and hallucinations can be seen in patients with hyperthyroidism

---

DIRECTIONS (Questions 60 and 61): Each group of questions below consists of lettered headings followed by a list of numbered words, phrases, or statements. For each numbered word, phrase, or statement, select the ONE lettered heading that is most closely associated with it. Each lettered heading may be selected once, more than once, or not at all.

  A. auditory hallucinations and pressured speech with delusions
  B. pressured speech without delusions
  C. slowed speech and loss of interests in hobbies
  D. early morning awakening with unrefreshing sleep

60. Manic episode with psychotic features

61. Manic episode without psychotic features

DIRECTIONS (Questions 62 through 101): Each group of questions below consists of lettered headings followed by a list of numbered words, phrases, or statements. For each numbered word, phrase, or statement, select the ONE lettered heading that is most closely associated with it. Each lettered heading may be selected once, more than once, or not at all.

Questions 62 through 66

    A. judgment
    B. memory
    C. affect
    D. insight
    E. perception

62. Remembering words

63. "What would you do if you were lost in the woods without a compass?"

64. Observable manifestation of mood

65. "How do you understand the problems that brought you here?"

66. "Please try to name the last three presidents"

Questions 67 through 71

    A. delirium
    B. dementia
    C. compulsion
    D. akathisia
    E. waxy flexibility

67. Gradual deterioration from a previous level of intellectual functioning with clear consciousness

68. Compelling urge that one fights against

69. Rapid onset of agitation or stupor with clouded consciousness

70. Limb is moveable with resistance but stays in the position into which it is moved

71. Subjective anxiety with objective fidgetiness

Questions 72 through 76

    A. Minnesota Multiphasic Personality Inventory–2 (MMPI–2)
    B. Thematic Apperception Test (TAT)
    C. Rorschach
    D. Wechsler Adult Intelligence Scale–Revised (WAIS–R)
    E. Halstead–Reitan

72. The patient tells stories based on pictures

73. Neuropsychological battery

74. Empirically based personality test

75. Verbal and performance tasks

76. Projective test using abstract visual stimuli

Questions 77 through 81

    A. cocaine intoxication
    B. cocaine withdrawal
    C. alcohol intoxication
    D. alcohol withdrawal
    E. heroin withdrawal

77. Nausea, vomiting, abdominal cramps, and muscle pain

78. Leading cause of traffic offenses

79. Formication

80. Seizures, cardiovascular collapse, and death

81. Severe depression

Questions 82 through 86

    A. schizophrenia
    B. mania
    C. depression
    D. antisocial personality disorder
    E. alcoholism

82. Euphoric or irritable mood

83. Onset of symptoms before age 15

84. Higher prevalence among women

85. Self-help groups help provide most treatment

86. Dementia praecox

Questions 87 through 91

    A. single photon emission computed tomography (SPECT)
    B. brain electrical activity mapping (BEAM)
    C. positron emission tomography (PET)
    D. magnetic resonance imaging (MRI)
    E. computed tomography (CT)

87. Involves no exposure to radiation or powerful electromagnetic fields

88. Imaging procedure of choice for a 50-year-old man with a metal plate in his skull who suffers major head trauma

89. Useful in visualizing the posterior fossa

90. Requires a cyclotron

91. Permits visualization of the brain performing functions that occur in milliseconds

Questions 92 through 96

    A. paranoid schizophrenia
    B. catatonic schizophrenia
    C. disorganized schizophrenia
    D. residual schizophrenia
    E. undifferentiated schizophrenia

92. Also called hebephrenic schizophrenia

93. Characterized by delusions of persecution or grandeur

94. Onset often occurs in the late twenties or early thirties

95. Patients can alternate between stupor and excitement

96. Patients currently show no prominent psychotic symptoms

Questions 97 through 101

    A. seen only in men
    B. seen only in women
    C. seen more frequently in men
    D. seen more frequently in women
    E. seen equally frequently in both sexes

97. Huntington's disease

98. Major depression

99. Bipolar I disorder

100. Alcohol abuse

101. Schizophrenia

Diagnosis and Evaluation

Explanatory Answers

1. (D) The patient should feel that you are concerned and interested in *her,* not her symptoms. While she may well be depressed or have a somatization disorder or hypochondriasis, it is much too abrupt to tell her she should see a psychiatrist. She will likely feel discounted and think that you are telling her "nothing is wrong" with her or that "it is all in her head" when she knows she is suffering. (**Ref. 6,** pp. 31–34)

2. (E) Personal history is not part of the mental status examination. Indeed, the mental status examination is a description of a person's mental status at one point and time—much like the "still pictures" advertising a movie. The mental status exam does not tell where the person has been or where he is going. (**Ref. 6,** pp. 37–40)

3. (C) The psychosocial formulation brings together all the factors—biological, psychological, and sociocultural—that explain why a patient is ill in this way at this time. It provides a conceptual framework for treatment. (**Ref. 2,** pp. 92–96)

4. (D) The performance scale of the WAIS–R includes problems requiring reproducing designs with blocks. Arithmetic and similarities are in verbal subtexts. (**Ref. 2,** pp. 126–127)

5. (E) The WAIS–R is a test of intelligence, but is influenced by culture and achievement. It includes both verbal and performance subtests. Various patterns among subtests may be of use in differentiating different types of psychopathology. (**Ref. 2,** pp. 126– 127)

6. (D) The subject makes up a story for each of several pictures. The TAT is a projective test. It is believed the subject will read into the pictures themes and conflicts important in his inner life. (**Ref. 2,** pp. 135–136)

7. (C) If erections occur in a man while he is asleep, a psychological cause of impotence is likely. Other useful tests to rule out an organic cause are measuring penile blood pressure and testing pudendal nerve latency time. (**Ref. 6,** p. 360)

8. (E) The Rorschach (inkblot) is a projective test. All the other tests noted are used to detect organic mental illness. However, it should be noted that skilled interpreters can use almost any test to infer information. Because of that, the physician is wise to tell the psychologist interpreting the test what information he wishes to know. (**Ref. 2,** pp. 134–135)

9. (E) The reduced metabolic rate induced by starvation is accompanied by hypotension, *not* hypertension. Hypothermia, dependent edema, bradycardia, and lanugo hair are other signs of starvation. (**Ref. 6,** p. 378)

10. (B) Extreme wakefulness may be a sign of sedative–hypnotic withdrawal, but not of sedative–hypnotic intoxication. Sleepiness (or even stupor) is seen in sedative–hypnotic intoxication. (**Ref. 6,** pp. 314–317)

11. (B) "Ice" is a crystallized form of methamphetamine. It has recently caused considerable social problems, particularly in Hawaii. (**Ref. 6,** p. 320)

12. (B) All of the named groups follow 12-step programs to help recovering patients share their experiences. As implied by its name, however, Overeaters Anonymous is comprised largely of patients with obesity or eating disorders, while the other groups consist of alcohol and drug abusers. (**Ref. 6,** p. 329)

13. **(C)** SPECT is the acronym for single photon emission computed tomography. SPECT allows measurement of cerebral metabolism and blood flow at a moment in time. **(Ref. 6,** p. 146)

14. **(D)** Catalepsy is a state of immobility. Waxy flexibility describes the characteristic of patients to hold a body part in a position in which it is placed. Automatism is automatic and apparently undirected motor behavior that is not consciously controlled; stereotypy is the persistent, mechanical repetition of speech or motor activity. Reaction formation, on the other hand, is a Freudian defense mechanism involving the adoption of attitudes that are the exact opposite of unacceptable impulses. **(Ref. 5,** pp. 37, 220)

15. **(C)** Although the dexamethasone suppression test can provide useful corollary information about the presence of depression, it has low sensitivity and specificity and there are frequent false-positive and false-negative results. A positive or abnormal response is characterized by a failure of serum cortisol levels to be reduced the day after the administration of oral dexamethasone. **(Ref. 2,** p. 124)

16. **(D)** There are many organic causes of mental disorder. Vitamin deficiency, liver disease, and pneumonia can all cause abnormal mental states. A chest x-ray would be more useful than a bronchoscopy in the diagnosis of pneumonia in an individual with an organic mental disorder. **(Ref. 6,** p. 147)

17. **(D)** Bulimia is the episodic, uncontrolled gorging of large quantities of food in short periods of time. Most bulimic patients purge themselves and cause physical damage to themselves by frequent vomiting. All of the signs listed are typical of vomiting-induced signs except for the absence of a patellar reflex, which is not usually found in bulimia. **(Ref. 2,** pp. 331–333)

18. **(D)** Schizophrenia has a better prognosis in married patients who have had an acute onset of an illness with affective symptoms or a clouded sensorium and who have no family history of schizophrenia. Patients with a positive family history of schizophrenia, however, fall into the poor-prognosis group of schizophrenic patients. **(Ref. 6,** pp. 168–169)

19. (E) Many organic conditions and stimulant intoxication mimic schizophrenia. However, heroin intoxication presents as lethargy and is unlikely to be mistaken for schizophrenia. (Ref. 6, p. 169)

20. (D) A minority of depressed patients present with auditory hallucinations related to their mood. Visual hallucinations, on the other hand, are rare in depression. (Ref. 6, p. 196)

21. (A) It is essential that physicians learn to take a sexual history without undue shame or embarrassment. Patients will detect anxiety in their doctors, which will only serve to increase their own anxiety. (Ref. 6, pp. 357–362)

22. (A) In 1973, the American Psychiatric Association voted to remove homosexuality from its list of mental disorders. It is now considered a sexual disorder only if it is unacceptable to the patient, in which case the DSM–IV diagnosis is "sexual disorder not otherwise specified." (Ref. 4, p. 538)

23. (D) Ten percent of schizophrenics commit suicide. It is important to keep the high suicide risk of schizophrenics in mind when evaluating them. (Ref. 6, p. 166)

24. (D) When paranoia, disorganization, or catatonic motor behavior predominate, they are the basis of subtypes of schizophrenia. Undifferentiated schizophrenia is not typified by predominance of one particular symptom. "Phlegmatic" is a literary term used to describe individuals who do not easily share their emotions. (Ref. 4, pp. 286–290)

25. (E) Positive symptoms of schizophrenia include hallucinations, delusions, bizarre behavior, and marked formal thought disorder. Flat affect, poverty of speech, apathy, and impaired hygiene are negative symptoms of schizophrenia. (Ref. 6, p. 164)

26. (A) PET scans are available only in a limited number of medical centers. PET involves the administration of a radioactive tracer that emits positrons and allows the visualization of metabolism. At the present time, PET scans are extremely expensive. (Ref. 6, pp. 93–94)

27. **(C)** MRIs generally provide better resolution than CTs but are more expensive. The risk of CT scans is of radiation exposure, whereas that of MRI scans is of exposure to a strong electromagnetic field. Because of the strength of the electromagnetic field, MRI scans are contraindicated in patients with implanted cardiac pacemakers. **(Ref. 6,** pp. 80–88)

28. **(D)** SPECT provides a direct measure of cerebral blood flow. As the symptoms of AIDS dementia begin, patients suffering from the illness typically begin to develop patchy areas of decreased perfusion on SPECT scans. **(Ref. 6,** p. 92)

29. **(B)** Men attempt suicide much less frequently than women but complete it more frequently. Other characteristics of suicide completers are older age, schizophrenic diagnoses, careful planning, and acting when help is unavailable. **(Ref. 6,** p. 398)

30. **(E)** A study done in New York showed that the suicide rate in AIDS patients is nearly 60 times that of the general population. Five percent of suicide completers have serious physical illnesses at the time of the suicide. **(Ref. 6,** pp. 394–395)

31. **(D)** Hypertension is seen frequently in acute PCP intoxication. The drug is similar to ketamine and can cause severe toxic side effects, including psychosis and coma. **(Ref. 5,** pp. 428–430)

32. **(C)** The Bender gestalt test is a simple test for organic mental disorders which requires individuals to copy nine geometric patterns. Most people can draw the figures without difficulty, and problems with the task may indicate a perceptual or motor problem. **(Ref. 2,** p. 127)

33. **(E)** Anticholinergic medication frequently increases the agitation of demented persons. On the other hand, a low-stimulus environment, consistency, and the treatment of accompanying psychiatric problems tend to be clinically useful for them. **(Ref. 6,** pp. 148–149)

34. **(D)** Huntington's disease is transmitted by a dominant gene on chromosome 4. Hence, about one-half of the offspring of an individual with the illness will inherit the disease. **(Ref. 6,** p. 148)

35. (C) Persons with an IQ under 70 are considered mentally retarded. Their IQs are more than two standard deviations below the population mean. (**Ref. 6,** pp. 442–443)

36. (B) Depressed patients typically show "reduced REM latency." They show a shorter time from the onset of sleep until the first REM period. (**Ref. 5,** pp. 160–161)

37. (A) 15% of women in a study of "normal couples" reported a total inability to have orgasms. Eleven percent of women in such couples reported that they reach orgasms too quickly. (**Ref. 6,** p. 358)

38. (D) Of men in a study of "normal couples," 36% complained that they ejaculate too quickly. Four percent of men in such couples complained of difficulty ejaculating. (**Ref. 6,** p. 358)

39. (A) Vaginismus is the involuntary contraction of the outer vagina, preventing intercourse. Dyspareunia is pain on intercourse. (**Ref. 6,** p. 359)

40. (C) Approximately 3% of children are mentally retarded. Six million children and adults in the U.S. are mentally retarded. (**Ref. 5,** p. 681)

41. (D) Of the mentally retarded, 80% are mildly retarded. Twelve percent of the total are moderately retarded (IQs from 30 to 49), and 8% are profoundly or severely retarded (IQs below 34). (**Ref. 5,** pp. 682–683)

42. (C) Pseudodementia is a presentation of depressive illness in which the patient complains of difficulty thinking but makes little effort to perform well on the mental status examination. It is important to recognize the illness because it is a treatable depression. (**Ref. 6,** p. 145)

43. (A) Koro is a nonpsychotic hysterical reaction that occurs in southeast Asia in epidemic form. Men may complain that their penises are retracting into their abdomens. It is a good example of a culture-bound psychiatric disorder. (**Ref. 4,** p. 846)

44. (B) Opiate intoxication causes pupillary constriction. However, it should be noted that severe opiate overdoses can result in near-terminal anoxia, which results in pupillary dilation. (**Ref. 6,** p. 318)

45. (D) Intravenous heroin use is a strong positive reinforcer because it creates a variety of pleasurable symptoms in the user. They include euphoria and an orgasmic sensation in the abdomen. (**Ref. 6,** p. 318)

46. (B) Clonidine provides good suppression of the autonomic signs of heroin withdrawal. Naloxone, an opiate antagonist, worsens the symptoms of heroin withdrawal. (**Ref. 6,** p. 319)

47. (A) Methadone is used to replace heroin because it has a longer half-life than heroin. Hence, its dosage may be decreased gradually without an abrupt change in blood methadone levels. (**Ref. 6,** pp. 318–319)

48. (C) The Rorschach (inkblot) test allows patients to put into their interpretation of the ink blots projections of what are thought to be aspects of their personalities. WAIS–R is an intelligence test; MMPI–2 is a nonprojective personality test; and Halstead–Reitan and Luria–Nebraska tests are neuropsychological test batteries. (**Ref. 2,** pp. 126–137)

49. (D) Histrionic personality disorder is a diagnostic term given to individuals who are often seductive in appearance and behavior and overly concerned with physical attractiveness. Such individuals are often rather shallow in their emotions, despite their dramatic displays. (**Ref. 6,** pp. 334–348)

50. (A) A cardinal difference between avoidant and schizoid personality disorders is that persons with avoidant personality disorder long for human contact but fear it, whereas those with schizoid personality disorder seem indifferent towards it. The other personality disorders listed are linked with characteristics quite the opposite of expected in persons with those disorders. (**Ref. 2,** pp. 281–305)

51. (C) By screening infants at birth, individuals with phenylketonuria can be identified and prescribed a diet low in phenylalanine. By that means, their development of retardation can be avoided. **(Ref. 2,** p. 364)

52. (D) It is important for the psychiatric interviewer to establish rapport with the patient and to give the patient a chance to answer open-ended questions. It is also important not to feel defensive while interviewing. **(Ref. 6,** pp. 31–34)

53. (E) This patient demonstrates an active libido. Reduced sexual interest, on the other hand, is common during depression. **(Ref. 5,** p. 312)

54. (E) There is no evidence that this man suffers from auditory hallucinations, which are typical in psychotic disorders. He displays the defense mechanism of projection by placing some of the blame for his difficulty on the examining student. His impulsiveness and self-destructive, as well as antisocial, behavior point toward the presence of a personality disorder. **(Ref. 5,** pp. 221–222; **Ref. 6,** pp. 333–354)

55. (C) Wilson's disease is an autosomal recessive disorder of copper metabolism, which is manifested by hepatic, neurological, and psychiatric symptoms. Its age of onset generally is between 8 and 20 years, and it can be treated with dietary copper restrictions and d-penicillamine therapy. **(Ref. 1,** p. 111)

56. (E) Hypothyroidism usually causes weight gain and a deeper voice. Thin, dry hair; paranoia and depression; or hypomania can occur. **(Ref. 1,** p. 371)

57. (C) Absorption of alcohol is fastest from drinks containing 15% to 30% alcohol—that is 30- to 60-proof alcohol. **(Ref. 1,** p. 400)

58. (B) Caffeine withdrawal syndrome causes headaches and decreased alertness, which generally reach peak intensity 24 to 48 hours after the last dose of caffeine. Caffeine is a weak reinforcer in laboratory studies. Tolerance occurs to caffeine intake; 20% to 30% of adult Americans consume more than 500 milligrams of caffeine a day. **(Ref. 1,** pp. 416–419)

59. **(C)** Hyperthyroidism, which can be mimicked by exogenous thyroid hormones, typically presents with insomnia, rapid speech, and difficulty with concentration and memory. Surprisingly, energy levels often are subjectively decreased in patients with hyperthyroidism. (**Ref. 1,** pp. 371, 987–988)

60. **(A)** Auditory hallucinations can occur in patients with schizophrenia or in patients with a manic episode with psychotic features. In the case of a manic episode, the content of the hallucination is likely to be congruent with the patient's mood disturbance. (**Ref. 6,** p. 217)

61. **(B)** Both schizophrenia and manic episodes may present with disorganized speech reflective of a thought disorder. The differential diagnosis of schizophrenia from mania is a difficult and important one to make, as the treatment for the disorders may be quite different. Some manic episodes show increased psychomotor activity without psychotic features. Slowed speech and unrefreshing sleep are typical of depression, not mania. (**Ref. 6,** p. 217)

62. **(B)** Recent memory can be tested by asking a patient to remember several unrelated words. Poor attention can also make it difficult to remember words. (**Ref. 2,** p. 114)

63. **(A)** Practical judgment can be assessed by asking a patient how he would behave in a hypothetical situation. Its assessment is especially important in the evaluation of thought disorders, personality disorders, and dementia. (**Ref. 2,** p. 115)

64. **(C)** Affect is the observable correlate of emotion. It is shown by facial expression, gestures, and speech. (**Ref. 2,** pp. 111–112)

65. **(D)** A patient's degree of understanding of his medical or psychological problems is a measure of his insight. Poor insight may reflect a cognitive deficit or may be evidence of a psychodynamic defense. (**Ref. 2,** p. 116)

66. **(B)** Remote memory can be tested by asking factual questions. The average patient should know the answer to those questions, and the answer should be verifiable. (**Ref. 2,** p. 114)

67. **(B)** Dementia is characterized by an insidious onset with a normal level of arousal but a progressive impairment in mental functioning. (**Ref. 6,** p. 145)

68. **(C)** A compulsion is the need to repeat some action in a ritualistic manner, uncontrollable by an act of will. Sometimes, the action has a symbolic meaning. (**Ref. 2,** pp. 477–478)

69. **(A)** Delirium is a clouding of consciousness with the rapid onset of agitation or stupor. It is often reversible. (**Ref. 6,** p. 145)

70. **(E)** Waxy flexibility is a catatonic symptom in which the examiner encounters resistance upon attempting to move parts of a patient's body. However, once moved, they then remain in the position in which they are placed. (**Ref. 2,** p. 477)

71. **(D)** Akathisia is a side effect of neuroleptic antipsychotic medications. It causes patients to report that they feel compelled to pace or tap their feet. (**Ref. 6,** p. 481)

72. **(B)** The thematic apperception test (TAT) consists of a series of drawings shown to the patient, who is then asked to make up a story about the picture, presumably projecting his own personality through the story. (**Ref. 2,** pp. 135–136)

73. **(E)** The Halstead–Reitan battery is used for detailed neuropsychological testing. It can give valuable information about brain damage. (**Ref. 2,** pp. 128–129)

74. **(A)** The Minnesota Multiphasic Personality Inventory–2 (MMPI–2) consists of a large number of statements to which the patient answers "true" or "false." Personality profiles have been empirically constructed from responses to the questions. (**Ref. 2,** pp. 132–134)

75. **(D)** The Wechsler Adult Intelligence Scale–Revised (WAIS–R) is an IQ test that includes verbal and performance subtests. The subtests can help screen for organic deficits. (**Ref. 2,** pp. 126–127)

76. (C) The Rorschach inkblot test allows patients to project their feelings through their interpretation of abstract inkblots. It requires sophisticated interpretation of the patients' responses in the light of their clinical presentations. (**Ref. 2,** pp. 134–135)

77. (E) Withdrawal from heroin or other potent opiates usually is not life threatening. It does cause severe unpleasant autonomic symptoms, as well as nausea, cramps, and muscle pain. (**Ref. 6,** p. 318)

78. (C) Alcohol intoxication, for the purpose of drunk driving offenses, is often defined as a blood alcohol concentration exceeding 100 milligrams per 100 milliliters of blood. One to one and one-half quarts of beer drunk in a short time can produce this blood level in an average adult. (**Ref. 5,** pp. 701–702)

79. (A) Formication is a tactile hallucination of insects crawling under the skin. It frequently occurs in cocaine intoxication. (**Ref. 5,** p. 40)

80. (D) Delirium tremens is the most severe form of alcohol withdrawal. Patients with delirium tremens, if left untreated, can die after seizures and cardiovascular collapse. (**Ref. 6,** p. 302)

81. (D) Severe depression can occur as cocaine abusers crash during withdrawal from the drug. Excessive sleep and overeating can also occur during cocaine withdrawal. (**Ref. 5,** pp. 420–422)

82. (B) Euphoria and grandiosity are most typical of mania of intermediate severity. Many severe manic episodes, on the other hand, are characterized by extreme irritability. (**Ref. 2,** pp. 226–229)

83. (D) DSM–IV criteria require a person to be 18 years old to be diagnosed as suffering from antisocial personality disorder. However, persons with the disorder have a history of pervasive antisocial behavior dating back to before age 15. (**Ref. 4,** pp. 645–650)

84. (C) The point prevalence of major depression is 2% to 3% for men. It is 5% to 9% for women. (**Ref. 4,** p. 341)

85. (E) Alcoholics Anonymous provides a worldwide network of self-help groups aimed at maintaining the sobriety of alcoholics through frequent meetings and other programs. Members give each other acceptance, understanding, forgiveness, and confrontation. (**Ref. 6,** p. 305)

86. (A) Dr. Emil Kraepelin, who is largely responsible for the understanding of the difference between schizophrenia and affective disorders, called schizophrenia "dementia praecox." The term "schizophrenia" was coined in the twentieth century by Dr. Eugen Bleuler. (**Ref. 6,** pp. 157–158)

87. (B) Brain electrical activity mapping (BEAM) provides two-dimensional maps of brain electrical activity generated by computer modification of EEG information. Its use in psychiatry is currently largely in researching mental illness. (**Ref. 6,** p. 80)

88. (E) Computed tomography (CT) allows visualization of brain tissue without exposing patients to the strong electromagnetic fields used in magnetic resonance imaging (MRI). A metal plate in the skull could be attracted to the powerful magnet of an MRI machine. (**Ref. 6,** pp. 81–85)

89. (D) Magnetic resonance imaging (MRI) allows good visualization of the posterior fossa. That area is difficult to see with a CT scan because of the density of bone in that region. (**Ref. 6,** p. 86)

90. (C) Positron emission tomography (PET) scans involve the injection of positron-emitting atoms with short half-lives which must be generated at a nearby cyclotron. This limits its geographic availability. (**Ref. 6,** p. 93)

91. (D) Brain electrical activity mapping (BEAM) is at present the only brain imaging technique that allows visualization of extremely short-term brain functions. It does so by integrating EEG information in extremely short time increments into a two-dimensional map of brain electrical activity. (**Ref. 6,** p. 80)

92. (C) Disorganized or hebephrenic schizophrenia is characterized by primitive, often silly, behavior. The affect is flat or inappropriate. (**Ref. 4,** pp. 287–288)

93. (A) Paranoid schizophrenia is characterized by delusions of persecution or grandeur. The delusions may be multiple but are usually organized around a coherent theme. (**Ref. 4,** p. 287)

94. (A) Paranoid schizophrenia has a later onset than other types. Patients with the disorder have often established a social life by the time of onset of the illness, which may help them through the illness. (**Ref. 1,** p. 471)

95. (B) Patients with catatonic schizophrenia may present with either catatonic stupor or catatonic excitement. They may alternate between those two states. (**Ref. 4,** pp. 288–289)

96. (D) Residual schizophrenia is a name used for patients who have had a previous episode of schizophrenia with psychosis but who show no prominent psychotic symptoms at the present evaluation. They often continue to show negative symptoms of schizophrenia. (**Ref. 4,** pp. 289–290)

97. (E) Huntington's disease is an autosomal dominant disorder. It occurs, on the average, in one-half of the boys and one-half of the girls with the gene. (**Ref. 1,** p. 1161)

98. (D) Major depression is more frequently seen in females than in males by a factor of two. There are no described racial differences in the prevalence of mood disorders. Lifetime risk for females is 10% to 25% in community samples. (**Ref. 4,** p. 341)

99. (E) Unlike major depression, bipolar I disorder is equally common in males and females. Bipolar I disorder differs from bipolar II disorder in that patients have at least one clearly manic episode rather than only hypomanic episodes. Bipolar II disorder, on the other hand, may be more common in women than in men. (**Ref. 4,** pp. 353, 360)

100. (C) At all ages, up to five times more males than females are heavy drinkers. However, alcohol abuse tends to develop later in life in females. (**Ref. 4,** pp. 201–202)

101. (E) Community-based prevalence studies indicate that schizophrenia is equally common in both sexes. Lifetime prevalence is approximately 1.3%. It is important to note, though, that some hospital-based studies suggest a higher rate for males. (**Ref. 1,** p. 458; **Ref. 4,** pp. 281–282)

4

Mental Disorders and DSM–IV

John E. Pappenheim
Elizabeth Caspary

DIRECTIONS (Questions 1 through 59): Each of the questions or incomplete statements below is followed by five suggested answers or completions. Select the ONE that is best in each case.

---

1. Phencyclidine psychosis is characterized by all of the following EXCEPT
   A. hallucinations
   B. unpredictable assaultiveness
   C. paranoia
   D. clouded sensorium
   E. restlessness

2. Depressive "pseudodementia" is BEST differentiated from dementia by
   A. loss of remote memory
   B. illusions
   C. retained higher cortical function
   D. halting gait
   E. poor impulse control

3. Amnestic syndrome may be characterized by all of the following EXCEPT
   A. inability to learn new information
   B. inability to remember
   C. clouding of consciousness
   D. evidence of organic etiology
   E. retention of major intellectual abilities

4. Delusional disorder is characterized by
   A. clear consciousness
   B. loss of intellectual abilities
   C. loose associations
   D. bizarre behavior
   E. hallucinations

5. Symptoms of acute cocaine poisoning include all of the following EXCEPT
   A. anxiety
   B. paranoid ideation
   C. hallucinations
   D. tachycardia
   E. hypothermia

6. Which of the following must be present for a diagnosis of intoxication due to alcohol?
   A. loquacity
   D. slurred speech
   C. euphoria
   D. fighting
   E. none of the above

7. Which of the following is NOT a DSM–IV syndrome produced by alcohol?
   A. alcohol-induced psychotic disorder
   B. alcohol withdrawal delirium
   C. alcohol intoxication delirium
   D. alcohol-induced mood disorder
   E. alcohol-induced paraphilia

8. Alcohol hallucinosis is characterized by all of the following EXCEPT
   A. auditory hallucinations
   B. occurrence within two days of alcohol withdrawal
   C. voices that may discuss the person in the third person
   D. close relation to prominent delusions
   E. duration of several weeks

9. When a person suffers from a slowly progressing nonaffective psychotic disorder, lasting longer than 6 months, but there is insufficient information to make a diagnosis of schizophrenic disorder, the BEST diagnosis is
   A. atypical psychosis (psychotic disorder, NOS)
   B. brief psychotic disorder
   C. schizophreniform disorder
   D. schizoaffective disorder
   E. pervasive developmental disorder

10. Paraphilias are characterized by all of the following EXCEPT
    A. repetitiveness
    B. compulsion
    C. patterned nature of the activity
    D. symbolic substitutive satisfaction
    E. high rate of retrograde ejaculation with orgasm

11. Which of the following statements is NOT true of anorexia nervosa?
    A. there is an intense fear of gaining weight or becoming fat
    B. the mortality rate is 5% to 15%
    C. it is predominant a disorder of females
    D. it is always accompanied by bulimia
    E. in females, there is the presence of primary or secondary amenorrhea

12. The DSM-IV classification of mood disorders encompasses all of the following EXCEPT
    A. bipolar disorder
    B. dysthymia
    C. posttraumatic stress disorder
    D. cyclothymia
    E. major depression

13. Which of the following statements is TRUE of dysthymic disorder?
   A. symptoms are less intense and pervasive than major depression
   B. symptoms have characteristics of both depressive and manic syndromes
   C. hypomanic features must be of at least two years duration
   D. it is a variety of bipolar disorder
   E. none of the above statements are true

14. Which of the following statements is NOT true of bipolar disorder?
   A. it occurs in 0.4% to 1.2% of the general adult population
   B. it has a familial pattern associated with it
   C. the first episode usually occurs between 20 and 40 years of age
   D. depression occurs more frequently than mania
   E. forty percent of patients with typical bipolar disorder respond to lithium

15. The concept of uncomplicated bereavement includes all of the following EXCEPT
   A. it is not a mental disorder under DSM-IV
   B. it is not categorized as a major depressive episode under DSM-IV
   C. it is a normal reaction
   D. it is of varied duration among different cultural groups
   E. it is an exacerbation of a previous mental disorder

16. All of the following are characteristic of melancholia EXCEPT
   A. loss of interest or pleasure in all or almost all activities
   B. lack of reactivity to pleasurable stimuli
   C. depression regularly worse in the morning
   D. endogenous origin
   E. consistent early morning awakening

17. Which of the following statements is NOT true?
    A. fifty percent of individuals with major depression (single episode) have another major depressive episode sometime in their life
    B. the initial episode in bipolar disorders often is manic
    C. bipolar disorder depressive episodes generally are shorter than major unipolar depression
    D. twenty to thirty-five percent of individuals with the diagnosis of major depression (recurrent) will follow a chronic course
    E. major depressive episodes are never superimposed on dysthymic disorders

18. An individual whose symptomatology fulfills the criteria for dysthymic disorder but who has intermittent periods of normal mood which last more than a few months is BEST classified as having
    A. depressive disorder, not otherwise specified
    B. dysthymic disorder
    C. cyclothymic disorder
    D. major depressive episode
    E. none of the above

19. The bipolar I disorder classification is appropriate for patients with each of the following clinical presentations EXCEPT
    A. multiple manic episodes without depression
    B. current mania without prior affective disturbance
    C. current mania with prior depressive episodes
    D. recurrent depressions without prior mania
    E. recurrent depressions with prior mania

20. Under the DSM-IV classification, postconcussional disorder is characterized by all of the following EXCEPT
    A. fatigability
    B. disordered sleep
    C. categorization as a research criteria set
    D. enuresis
    E. decreased attention or memory

21. Delusions belong in the group of
    A. perceptual disorders
    B. behavioral disorders
    C. thought content disorders

    D. thought process disorders

    E. disturbances of affective response

22. Amphetamine-induced psychotic disorder is characterized by all of the following EXCEPT

    A. visual and/or tactile hallucinations

    B. ideas of reference

    C. persecutory delusions

    D. a clear state of consciousness

    E. early morning awakening

23. Posttraumatic stress disorder is characterized by all of the following EXCEPT

    A. reexperiencing of traumatic events

    B. numbing of responsiveness

    C. excessive autonomic arousal

    D. impairment of memory or concentration

    E. thought insertion

24. Dissociative disorders include all of the following EXCEPT

    A. amnesia

    D. fugue

    C. multiple personality

    D. depersonalization disorder

    E. posttraumatic stress disorder

25. Substance dependence may refer to all of the following EXCEPT

    A. tolerance or withdrawal

    B. pattern of pathological use

    C. impairment of social or occupational functioning

    D. minimal duration of one month

    E. underlying personality disorder

26. Which of the following is under conscious control?

    A. conversion disorder

    B. somatization disorder

    C. psychogenic pain disorder

    D. factitious disorder with physical symptoms

    E. hypochondriasis

27. Adjustment disorder is characterized by all of the following EX-CEPT
    A. maladaptive reaction
    B. occurrence of stressor within previous three months
    C. exacerbation of mental disorder
    D. maladaptive reaction persisting for less than six months
    E. impairment in social or occupational functioning

28. Wernicke's encephalopathy is characterized by all of the following EXCEPT
    A. thiamine avitaminosis
    B. depression and anxiety
    C. paralysis of external ocular muscles
    D. memory loss
    E. beriberi

29. Which of the following statements regarding delirium is NOT true?
    A. it rarely persists over one month
    B. fluctuations in symptoms are common
    C. psychomotor activity is disturbed
    D. memory impairment is pathognomonic
    E. it frequently presents initially as profound dysphoria

30. Common perceptual disturbances in delirium are
    A. loosening of associations
    B. delusions
    C. hallucinations
    D. difficulty sustaining attention
    E. insomnia

31. Common neurological signs in delirium are
    A. tremor
    B. sixth nerve palsy
    C. autonomic signs
    D. Babinski sign
    E. snout reflex

32. Clouding of consciousness is NOT found in
    A. coma
    B. delirium

C. amnestic disorder
D. intoxication
E. postictal state

33. Which of the following statements is NOT true regarding alcohol intoxication?
   A. symptoms are more marked when blood level is rising
   B. death occurs at blood levels from 400 to 700 mg%
   C. most people become intoxicated at blood levels between 100 and 200 mg%, although some do at levels as low as 20 mg%
   D. signs of intoxication include slurred speech, ataxia, and nystagmus
   E. in general, the body can metabolize approximately two drinks an hour

34. Which of the following complications associated with alcohol intoxication is NOT accurately represented?
   A. more than one-half of all murders
   B. approximately one-half of all highway fatalities
   C. risk of developing subdural hematomas upon falling
   D. one-half of suicides
   E. death usually resulting from respiratory suppression or aspiration of vomitus

35. Which of the following is NOT diagnostic for alcohol idiosyncratic intoxications?
   A. aggressiveness
   B. malingering
   C. atypical behavior
   D. no recollection of the incident
   E. blood alcohol level under 100 mg/dL

36. Which of the following is NOT seen in uncomplicated alcohol withdrawal?
   A. weakness
   B. nausea or vomiting
   C. delirium
   D. autonomic hyperactivity, such as tachycardia, sweating, and hypertension
   E. depressed mood or irritability

37. Substance abuse is distinguished from nonpathological substance use by all of the following EXCEPT
    A. recurrent adverse consequences
    B. impaired social or occupational functioning
    C. duration of at least one month
    D. recurrent use in physically hazardous situations
    E. blatant disregard for the illegality of the substance being used

38. Chronic, pathological alcohol abuse may be evidenced by all of the following EXCEPT
    A. regular daily intake of large amounts
    B. sobriety interspersed with binges
    C. regular heavy drinking limited to weekends
    D. atypical aggressive behavior after minimal alcohol ingestion
    E. relatively minimal development of tolerance

39. In DSM–IV, classification of phobic disorders may be divided into all of the following categories EXCEPT
    A. social phobia
    B. specific phobia
    C. taphophobia
    D. agoraphobia without panic disorder
    E. agoraphobia with panic disorder

40. All of the following statements regarding agoraphobia are true EXCEPT
    A. it is most commonly seen without panic attacks
    B. it represents a state of extreme fear of being incapacitated in an open or public place and unable to find help
    C. the fear frequently is decreased when the patient is accompanied by a friend or relative
    D. patients tend to restrict their activities and excursions to increasingly smaller areas
    E. frequent fears include dizziness or falling, loss of bowel or bladder control, and cardiac distress

41. For schizophrenic patients, studies carried out in England and the United States have shown that the MOST powerful predictor of relapse in the nine months following discharge from an inpatient treatment setting has been
 A. maintenance on depot neuroleptic
 B. familial expressed emotion
 C. absence of auditory hallucinations
 D. stable nocturnal sleep cycle
 E. absence of tardive dyskinesia

42. Which one of the following statements is NOT true of the treatment of schizophrenic disorder?
 A. the best results in schizophrenics are obtained by the combination of psychosocial therapy, drug therapy, and a task-oriented psychological approach
 B. neuroleptics speed up the process of recovery for most patients
 C. neuroleptics reduce the risk of relapse
 D. depot neuroleptics may aid in compliance with some patients
 E. addition of lithium frequently augments the efficacy of neuroleptics, especially if depot

43. Kernberg believes all of the following are true of borderline personalities EXCEPT
 A. the borderline experiences people as "all good" or "all bad"
 B. the borderline uses projective identification
 C. the defense of splitting is used to keep separate the experience of the "good mother" and the experience of the "bad mother"
 D. the borderline patient sets up a "mirror transference"
 E. the borderline patient experiences good feelings only by a flight into omnipotence

44. Which of the following is unlikely to dominate the clinical picture in major depressive episodes?
 A. mood-incongruent delusions
 B. dysphoric mood
 C. suicidal ideation
 D. self-reproach
 E. early morning awakening

45. Uncomplicated bereavement is NOT characterized by
  A. preoccupation with worthlessness
  B. transient thoughts of guilt
  C. thoughts that the patient should have died with the loved one
  D. full depressive syndrome
  E. transient course of 1 to 6 months

46. Adjustment disorder with depressed mood is characterized by all of the following EXCEPT
  A. identifiable psychosocial stressor
  B. impairment in social or occupational functioning
  C. remission after stressor ceases
  D. exacerbation of another mental disorder
  E. feelings of hopelessness

47. Anorexia nervosa is characterized by all of the following EXCEPT
  A. intense fear of becoming obese
  B. weight loss of at least 25%
  C. disturbance of body image
  D. onset in early- to late-adolescence
  E. amenorrhea

48. Hypochondriasis is typified by all of the following EXCEPT
  A. unrealistic interpretations of physical sensations
  B. the fear of having a disease persists despite medical reassurance
  C. unrealistic fears
  D. somatic hallucinations
  E. duration of at least six months

49. Factors suggesting favorable prognosis for a child with infantile autism include
  A. normal fundoscopic exam
  B. interest in music
  C. development of meaningful language by age seven
  D. obsessive need for sameness
  E. head banging

50. Alcohol withdrawal delirium is characterized by all of the following EXCEPT
  A. onset within one week of abstinence
  B. onset after 5 to 15 years of heavy drinking
  C. acute psychotic reaction accompanied by autonomic hyperactivity or maladaptive behavior and fluctuating clouding of consciousness
  D. visual hallucinations
  E. elevated serum ammonia levels

51. "Clouding of consciousness" is characterized by all of the following EXCEPT
  A. reduction in awareness of environment
  B. difficulty in sustaining attention
  C. disorientation of person, place, and time
  D. primary process thinking
  E. olfactory hallucinations

52. Which of the following is NOT characteristic of cocaine addiction?
  A. physical withdrawal is characterized by pupillary dilatation
  B. prolonged use may lead to psychosis
  C. delusions of persecution and jealousy are common
  D. frequent occurrence of formicative paresthesias
  E. cessation produces dysphoria and fatigue

53. Dementia may be caused by all of the following EXCEPT
  A. toxic and metabolic disturbances
  B. brain trauma
  C. multiple infarcts
  D. HIV infection
  E. CNS deposition of amyloid-A

54. Klein-Levin syndrome is characterized by
  A. periodic hypersomnia
  B. anorexia
  C. trichotillomania
  D. sexual immaturity
  E. kleptomania

55. For a DSM–IV diagnosis of schizophrenia, loosening or incoherence of associations must be associated with one or more of the following EXCEPT
  A. flat or grossly inappropriate affect
  B. delusions
  C. social isolation or withdrawal
  D. hallucinations
  E. catatonic behavior

56. DSM–IV is what type of classification?
  A. categorical
  B. phonetic
  C. dimensional
  D. reflective
  E. integral

57. According to DSM–IV, dementia of the Alzheimer's type may be categorized as any of the following EXCEPT
  A. uncomplicated
  B. with delirium
  C. with hallucinations
  D. with delusions
  E. with depressed mood

58. Compared with the general population, who is more likely to develop dementia of the Alzheimer's type (early onset)?
  A. parents
  B. first-degree biological relatives
  C. sexual partners
  D. first cousins
  E. neighbors

59. In alcohol intoxication, one or more of the following signs develop during or shortly after alcohol ingestion EXCEPT
  A. slurred speech
  B. unsteady gait
  C. giggling
  D. nystagmus
  E. impairment in attention or memory

DIRECTIONS (Questions 60 through 111): Each group of questions below consists of lettered headings followed by a list of numbered words, phrases, or statements. For each numbered word, phrase, or statement, select the ONE lettered heading that is most closely associated with it. Each lettered heading may be selected once, more than once, or not at all.

Questions 60 through 68

    A. amnestic disorder
    B. Rett's disorder
    C. delirium
    D. dementia
    E. schizophrenia
    F. substance-induced mood disorder
    G. cocaine intoxication

60. Global cognitive impairment without clouding of consciousness

61. Fluctuating level of consciousness

62. Recurrent hallucinations, affective flattening

63. Manic symptomatology

64. Inability to learn new information

65. Reserpine

66. Associated with mental retardation

67. Methyldopa

68. Positive and negative symptoms for six months

Questions 69 through 71

    A. focal neurological signs (excluding aphasia)
    B. auditory hallucinations
    C. erotomania
    D. gradual, progressive deterioration

  69. Alcohol hallucinosis

  70. Primary degenerative dementia

  71. Multi-infarct dementia

Questions 72 through 74

    A. preferential use of inanimate objects for sexual gratification
    B. discomfort with anatomic sex
    C. cross-dressing for sexual excitement

  72. Transsexualism

  73. Fetishism

  74. Transvestic fetishism

Questions 75 through 77

    A. loss or alteration in physical functioning due to psychological factors
    B. presence of at least 8 symptoms; onset before age 30
    C. single major symptom; at times psychological factors may be etiologically involved in the symptoms

  75. Somatization disorder

  76. Conversion disorder

  77. Pain disorder

Questions 78 through 80: Some depression, following loss, may take different forms at different ages. Match the following.

    A. evident in prepuberty
    B. evident in adolescent boys
    C. evident in the elderly

78. Separation anxiety

79. Conduct disturbances

80. Pseudodementia

Questions 81 and 82

    A. two-year history of chronic, mild depression, characterized by loss of interest in pleasure
    B. two-year history of periods of mild depression and hypomania

81. Cyclothymic disorder

82. Dysthymic disorder

Questions 83 through 88

    A. pattern occurring within a 12-month period
    B. persistent concern for at least 1 month
    C. continuous signs for at least 6 months
    D. at least 1 week
    E. symptoms nearly every day for at least 2 weeks
    F. longer than 6 months without symptoms

83. Substance abuse disorder

84. Panic disorder

85. Schizophrenia

86. Delusional disorder

87. Major depressive episode

88. Posttraumatic stress disorder (delayed)

Questions 89 and 90

    A. fear of being alone
    B. fear of helplessness upon incapacitation
    C. fear of scrutiny and embarrassment
    D. fear of having a serious disease

89. Agoraphobia

90. Social phobia

Questions 91 through 96

    A. persistent violation of societal norms
    B. developmentally inappropriate impulsivity and activity
    C. continuous refusal to talk, at least to certain people
    D. disobedient, provocative opposition to authority figures
    E. distortions in the development of multiple, basic psychological functions
    F. lack of responsiveness to others; usually develops before 36 months of age

91. Attention-deficit hyperactivity disorder

92. Conduct disorder

93. Selective mutism

94. Oppositional–defiant disorder

95. Pervasive developmental disorder

96. Infantile autism

Questions 97 through 102

    A. REM sleep
    B. predominantly during stage I and REM sleep
    C. predominantly during stage II sleep
    D. during both stages III and IV sleep
    E. during both REM and non-REM sleep

97. Sleep terror disorder

98. Sleepwalking disorder

99. Sleep nightmare

100. Functional enuresis

101. Sleep-related bruxism

102. Nocturnal penile tumescence

Questions 103 through 106

    A. delirium
    B. dementia

103. Reduction in clarity of awareness of environment (essential feature)

104. Frequent illusions and hallucinations

105. Course usually chronic and deteriorating

106. Alzheimer's type most common form

Questions 107 through 111

    A. disorder in thought process
    B. disorder in thought content

107. Circumstantiality

108. Delusions

109. Word salad

110. Obsessions

111. Neologisms

DIRECTIONS (Questions 112 through 124): Each of the questions or incomplete statements below is followed by five suggested answers or completions. Select the ONE that is best in each case.

---

112. Which of the following is NOT true regarding the paranoid personality?
    A. delusions always present
    B. pervasive suspiciousness
    C. restricted affectivity
    D. hypersensitivity
    E. overconcern with hidden motives

113. The schizotypal personality disorder may show all of the following characteristics EXCEPT
    A. magical thinking
    B. ideas of reference
    C. recurrent illusions
    D. paranoid ideation
    E. delusions of thought insertion

114. The passive–aggressive personality is characterized by all of the following EXCEPT
    A. indirect resistance to demands for adequate performance
    B. longstanding social and occupational ineffectiveness

    C. diagnosis early in childhood
    D. procrastination
    E. intentional inefficiency

115. The dependent personality shows all of the following characteristics EXCEPT
    A. preoccupation with details
    B. avoidance of taking responsibility for self
    C. allowing others to assume responsibility
    D. higher prevalence rate in women
    E. discomfort when alone

116. In children, all of the following may be listed on Axis I, DSM–IV EXCEPT
    A. reading disorder
    B. mental retardation
    C. mathematics disorder
    D. disorder of written expression
    E. learning disorder, not otherwise specified (NOS)

117. Consider these symptoms: rigidity of behavioral patterns, hypersensitivity to criticism; blaming others for one's problems, and chronic suspiciousness. These symptoms BEST describe the
    A. paranoid personality disorder
    B. antisocial personality disorder
    C. histrionic personality disorder
    D. borderline personality disorder
    E. narcissistic personality disorder

118. According to the Kinsey study (1948), what percentage of adult males are homosexual?
    A. 1%
    B. 3.0%
    C. 5.0%
    D. 10.0%
    E. 15.0%

119. All the following are categories of sexual disfunction (DSM–IV) EXCEPT
- **A.** sexual desire disorder
- **B.** ego-dystonic homosexuality
- **C.** sexual arousal disorder
- **D.** orgasm disorder
- **E.** substance-induced sexual dysfunction disorder

120. Which of the following is not TRUE of dyspareunia?
- **A.** recurrent genital pain occurring before, during, or after intercourse
- **B.** marked distress or interpersonal difficulty
- **C.** more common in men than women
- **D.** not due exclusively to the direct effect of drug abuse
- **E.** not caused exclusively by a lack of lubrication

121. Of men treated for sexual disorders, approximately what percent are estimated to have premature ejaculations as a chief complaint?
- **A.** 5%
- **B.** 20%
- **C.** 35%
- **D.** 50%
- **E.** 75%

122. Which of the following personality disorders is MOST likely to appear eccentric or odd?
- **A.** schizotypal
- **B.** compulsive
- **C.** antisocial
- **D.** dependent
- **E.** borderline

123. Which of the following characteristics is NOT typical of the antisocial personality?
- **A.** history of conduct disorder before age 15
- **B.** impulsivity
- **C.** current age of at least 18
- **D.** grandiose sense of self-importance
- **E.** lack of remorse

124. In developmental reading disorder, the essential feature is a significant impairment in reading skills. This disorder may be caused by
  A. mental retardation
  B. inadequate schooling
  C. hearing defect
  D. attention-deficit hyperactivity disorder
  E. none of the above

DIRECTIONS (Questions 125 through 133): Each group of questions below consists of lettered headings followed by a list of numbered words, phrases, or statements. For each numbered word, phrase, or statement, select the ONE lettered heading that is most closely associated with it. Each lettered heading may be selected once, more than once, or not at all.

Questions 125 through 127

  A. dramatic
  B. eccentric
  C. anxious

125. Cluster A: Paranoid, schizoid, schizotypal

126. Cluster B: Histrionic, narcissistic, antisocial, borderline

127. Cluster C: Avoidant, dependent, compulsive

Questions 128 through 133

  A. deficit in capacity to form social relationships
  B. oddities of thought, perception, and speech
  C. grandiosity
  D. instability in many areas
  E. hypersensitivity to evaluation

128. Schizoid

129. Schizotypal

130. Histrionic

131. Narcissistic

132. Borderline

133. Avoidant

DIRECTIONS (Questions 134 through 169): Each of the questions or incomplete statements below is followed by five suggested answers or completions. Select the ONE that is best in each case.

---

134. When a person with borderline personality disorder finds himself or herself without a "holding" relationship, his/her affectual response is MOST likely to be
   A. sadness
   B. indifference
   C. panic
   D. dysphoria
   E. joy (secondary to reaction formation)

135. According to Margaret Mahler's theory of the borderline personality disorder, the disorder begins in which phase of development?
   A. symbiotic
   B. rapprochement
   C. differentiation
   D. consolidation and object constancy
   E. autistic

136. A patient suffering from obsessive–compulsive personality disorder who is generally high functioning is LEAST likely to employ which of the following defense mechanisms?
   A. isolation
   B. reaction formation
   C. repression
   D. splitting
   E. sublimation

137. Sigmund Freud described a triad of defense mechanisms as central features of the obsessive–compulsive personality. Which of the following is NOT part of that triad?
   A. undoing
   B. isolation
   C. denial
   D. reaction formation
   E. none of the above

138. An individual suffering from passive–aggressive personality disorder might be likely to express anger in all of the following ways EXCEPT
   A. verbal threats
   B. procrastination
   C. covert obstructionism
   D. stubbornness
   E. inefficiency

139. Which of the following is characteristic of the narcissistic personality disorder?
   A. views self as socially inept
   B. interpersonally exploitive
   C. unstable image of self
   D. preoccupied with detail
   E. none of the above

140. In "Dissociative Amnesia" (DSM–IV) (formerly "Psychogenic Amnesia" in DSM–IIIR), several types of memory disturbances are described that include all of the following EXCEPT
   A. localized
   B. systematized
   C. sporadic
   D. selective
   E. continuous

141. Dissociative fugue (formerly psychogenic fugue) (DSM–IV) is BEST differentiated from dissociative identity disorder (formerly multiple personality disorder) by
  A. travel away from home
  B. lack of repeated shifts of identity over time
  C. assumption of a completely new identity
  D. heavy alcohol use associated with fugue
  E. presence of olfactory hallucinations

142. According to DSM–IV, the essential feature of dissociative disorders is a disturbance in
  A. identity
  B. motor skills
  C. attention
  D. concentration
  E. orientation

143. All of the following statements are true of dissociative identity disorder EXCEPT
  A. each personality (identity) has patterns of perceiving and thinking that are similar across the various personalities
  B. it is usually considered the most serious of the dissociative disorders
  C. each personality may have a different handwriting style
  D. disturbance is not due to alcoholic blackouts
  E. at least two of the personalities take recurrent control of the person's behavior

144. Epidemiologic evidence and research believe which of the following statements to be TRUE about dissociative identity disorder?
  A. approximately 10% of all psychiatric patients have this disorder
  B. the disorder most commonly appears in the third decade
  C. there are no familial patterns of the disorder
  D. of persons with a diagnosed dissociative identity disorder, 60% are women and 40% are men
  E. a factor in the development of the disorder seems to be an absence of support from significant people

145. Which of the following is NOT categorized under dissociative disorders in DSM–IV?
   A. amnesia (psychogenic)
   B. identity disorder
   C. fugue (psychogenic)
   D. somnambulism
   E. depersonalization

146. DSM–IV criteria for anorexia nervosa includes all of the following EXCEPT
   A. intense fear of becoming fat
   B. weight maintenance at less than 85% of that expected for age and height
   C. disturbance in the perception of body image
   D. pattern of vigorous exercise to avoid weight gain
   E. amenorrhea (absence of at least three consecutive menstrual cycles)

147. In DSM–IV, all of the following are criteria for a diagnosis of bulimia EXCEPT
   A. fasting
   B. a sense of lack of control over eating
   C. misuse of diuretics
   D. binge eating occurring at least twice per week for 3 months
   E. absence of at least 3 consecutive menstrual periods

148. All of the following statements tend to be true about anorexia and bulimia EXCEPT
   A. eating binges usually involve high-carbohydrate, easily digested foods, such as ice cream, cookies, and breads
   B. remaining sexually attractive and sexually active is important
   C. bulimic patients usually find their symptoms more ego-dystonic than do anorectic patients
   D. mood disorders frequently may be found along with anorexia or bulimia
   E. compulsive stealing occurs in both

149. All of the following statements are accurate regarding tics EX-
     CEPT that they are
     A. involuntary movements or vocalizations
     B. rapid, brief, and sudden
     C. recurrent, repetitive, and stereotypic
     D. experienced as irresistible but can be suppressed for varying
         lengths of time
     E. purposeful and are usually precipitated by appropriate social
         cues

150. All of the following statements are true of Tourette's syndrome
     EXCEPT
     A. both multiple motor and one or more vocal tics have been
         present at some time
     B. tics occur many times a day
     C. no genetic vulnerability has been demonstrated as an etio-
         logic factor
     D. onset occurs before age 18
     E. symptoms may return even after prolonged periods of remis-
         sion

151. All of the following statements regarding risk factors for bipolar I
     affective disorder are true EXCEPT
     A. they are equally prevalent in men and women
     B. they are equally prevalent among different races
     C. they are more common in higher socioeconomic groups
     D. the age of onset usually is in the early 20s
     E. there is strong evidence for genetic linkage and inheritance

152. All of the following are factors that point to a poor progression in
     Bipolar I disorders EXCEPT
     A. premorbid poor occupational status
     B. being female
     C. alcohol dependence
     D. interepisode depression feature
     E. all of the above

153. All of the following are seen in hypomania EXCEPT
     A. elevated, expansive mood
     B. pressured speech

   C. marked impairment in normal functioning
   D. excessive involvement in potentially dangerous activities
   E. racing thoughts

154. All of the following characteristics are DSM–IV criteria for mania EXCEPT
   A. delusions of aristocracy
   B. grandiosity
   C. decreased need for sleep
   D. flight of ideas
   E. excessive involvement in risky, pleasurable activities

155. Mania tends to be characterized by all of the following EXCEPT
   A. increased appetite
   B. weight loss
   C. increased libido
   D. compulsivity
   E. maniacal strength

156. Which of the following cognitive dysfunctions is NOT a major aspect of Aaron Beck's structured theory of depression?
   A. negative self-perception
   B. experiencing the world as a negative, demanding, and defeating place
   C. experiencing interpersonal relations as intrusive and frightening but necessary
   D. the expectation of continued hardship, suffering, deprivation, and failure
   E. expectation of punishment

157. All the following are symptoms of a major depression EXCEPT
   A. disorientation to time
   B. delusions involving cancer or AIDS
   C. failure to care for personal hygiene
   D. thought blocking
   E. overemphasis on the "bad" things of life

158. The following are characteristics of paranoid schizophrenia EXCEPT
   A. disorganized speech
   B. delusions of grandeur
   C. auditory hallucination
   D. later age of onset
   E. relative preservation of emotional response

159. Characteristics of mania include all of the following EXCEPT
   A. racing thoughts
   B. blocking
   C. distractibility
   D. impaired judgment
   E. clang associations with rhymes and puns

160. The four fundamental symptoms of schizophrenia that Eugene Bleuler defined include all of the following EXCEPT
   A. autism
   B. abnormal associations in thinking
   C. auditory hallucinations
   D. abnormal affect
   E. ambivalence

161. Of the different types of delusions that may occur in schizophrenia, which of the following is LEAST likely to occur?
   A. delusions of infidelity
   B. somatic delusions
   C. delusions of control
   D. bizarre delusions
   E. persecutory delusions

162. The DSM–IV subtypes of schizophrenia include all of the following EXCEPT
   A. paranoid
   B. catatonic
   C. disorganized (hebephrenic)
   D. simple
   E. residual

163. Positive symptoms of schizophrenia, associated with a favorable response to antipsychotic medication, include all of the following EXCEPT
A. delusions of persecution
B. hallucinations
C. bizarre behavior
D. apathy
E. delusions of grandeur

164. Of the following, which is the LEAST likely to be considered a prodromal sign of schizophrenia?
A. complaints of headache
B. interest in abstract ideas
C. unusual speech
D. thought blocking
E. decline in social functioning

165. An ocular abnormality frequently found in schizophrenics is
A. diplopia
B. nystagmus
C. saccades (rapid eye movements)
D. sluggish pupils
E. ptosis

166. Of schizophrenics, 40% attempt suicide and about 10% succeed. Potential risk factors include all of the following EXCEPT
A. college education
B. depression
C. chronic symptomatology
D. command hallucinations
E. young age

167. Schizophrenic patients frequently demonstrate an inability to understand or to create the usual emotional inflections in speech. This is termed
A. echolalia
B. neologism
C. monotony
D. aprosodia
E. verbigeration

168. According to DSM–IV, for the diagnosis of schizophrenia, psychotic symptoms in the active phase must be present for how long, unless successfully treated?
   A. one week
   B. two weeks
   C. one month
   D. two months
   E. six months

169. When classifying the course of schizophrenia using DSM–IV, all of the following categories may be used EXCEPT
   A. continuous
   B. episodic with interepisodic residual symptoms
   C. single episode in full remission
   D. residual
   E. single episode in full remission

DIRECTIONS (Questions 170 through 199): This section consists of clinical situations, each followed by a series of questions. Study each situation and select the ONE best answer to each question following it.

Questions 170 through 174

Mr. Jones, a 55-year-old married man, was brought to the hospital by his family because he was found wandering several miles from his home. Over the past year, he has become anxious and agitated. He is unable to keep his checkbook balanced. He has become quite compulsive, carefully putting articles in the same place; however, he often forgets where he puts things and accuses others of stealing them.

On admission, he was disheveled and agitated. He did not know where he was or how he had arrived. His recent memory was poor. He showed marked deterioration in general intellectual functions. He was unable to copy three-dimensional figures or to assemble blocks into specific designs. Physical examination was unremarkable, EXCEPT for some hyperreflexia. Laboratory studies were normal.

170. The MOST likely axis I diagnosis is
   A. dementia of the Alzheimer's type with early onset
   B. dementia of the Alzheimer's type with late onset
   C. multi-infarct dementia

    D. dementia with axis III diagnosis of myxedema

    E. dementia with axis III diagnosis of tertiary syphilis

171. The axis II diagnosis is
- **A.** dependent personality disorder
- **B.** compulsive personality disorder
- **C.** paranoid personality disorder
- **D.** schizoid personality disorder
- **E.** none of the above

172. Of the following, which is NOT characteristic of a cortical dementia?
- **A.** early aphasia
- **B.** impaired memory
- **C.** chorea
- **D.** early impairment of calculation skills
- **E.** upright posture

173. Axis V diagnosis, current global assessment of functioning (GAF), is approximately
- **A.** 10
- **B.** 35
- **C.** 55
- **D.** 70
- **E.** 20

174. Of the following, which is the MOST likely diagnosis?
- **A.** Pick's disease
- **B.** tertiary syphilis
- **C.** Alzheimer's disease
- **D.** myxedema
- **E.** normal pressure hydrocephalus

Questions 175 through 185

A 40-year-old white married woman comes to the clinic with complaints of vague abdominal pain of three months' duration and the certainty that she has cancer. She has been referred to the clinic after exhaustive medical examinations, the results of which have always been within normal limits. Despite numerous tests and hospitalizations, she continues to believe that she has cancer, but "the doctors just haven't found it yet."

Over the past three months, she has experienced early morning awakening and loss of appetite. She has lost 12 pounds, which she attributes to the effects of cancer. She is unable to find even momentary pleasure in anything and has been unable to do her housework. She thinks her family would be better off without her. She has a sad, fixed facies. Her speech is monotonous and slow. Her sentences often begin after long, sighing expirations. Tears come to her eyes when she begins to talk about the fact that her youngest child left for college three months ago.

Previously she had been well. She denies a previous history of similar symptoms and has received no prior medical or psychiatric help. Although regarded by others as unduly serious, formal, and perfectionistic, she takes pride in the way she is: "I guess I was a 'workaholic,' but that's the way I am."

175. Which of the following is the MOST likely axis I diagnosis?
- **A.** bipolar disorder
- **B.** schizoaffective disorder
- **C.** major depression (single episode)
- **D.** cancer of the pancreas
- **E.** hypochondriasis

176. Which of the following is the MOST likely axis II diagnosis?
- **A.** obsessive–compulsive personality disorder
- **B.** avoidant personality disorder
- **C.** compulsive traits
- **D.** borderline personality disorder
- **E.** no diagnosis on axis II

177. Which of the following would NOT be used to justify a subclassification of melancholia?
   A. significant weight loss
   B. anhedonia
   C. depression that is worse in the morning
   D. marked psychomotor retardation
   E. delusions of cancer

178. If the patient had a previous similar episode from which she completely recovered, the MOST probable diagnosis would be
   A. dysthymic disorder
   B. cyclothymic disorder
   C. bipolar disorder (depressed)
   D. atypical depression
   E. major depression (recurrent)

179. The patient's insistence that she has cancer despite normal medical work-ups and reassurance is an example of
   A. a somatic delusion
   B. phobia
   C. conversion
   D. psychophysiologic reaction
   E. none of the above

180. Patients with this disorder
   A. should not be asked about suicide
   B. should be asked about suicide
   C. rarely attempt suicide
   D. make manipulative gestures but rarely complete suicide
   E. are most likely to overdose, as opposed to using other means of suicide

181. During treatment, which of the following should make the therapist LESS concerned about suicide?
   A. the patient's mood and energy level improves
   B. the patient has a family history of suicide
   C. the patient tells about her suicidal ideas and plans, not disavowing them
   D. the patient made a suicidal gesture one week ago
   E. none of the above

182. Which of the following statements is NOT true of suicide?
    A. about 25,000 suicides are reported annually in the United States
    B. certified suicides constitute 12 deaths per 100,000
    C. men commit suicide three times more frequently than women
    D. among men, the rate of suicide peaks after age 45
    E. marriage increases the risk of suicide

183. From a psychoanalytic point of view, this patient can be conceptualized as fixated at or regressed to the
    A. oral stage
    B. anal stage
    C. separation–individual stage
    D. oedipal stage
    E. latency stage

184. The MOST appropriate pharmacotherapy would be
    A. desipramine
    B. haloperidol
    C. desipramine and haloperidol
    D. desipramine and diazepam
    E. haloperidol and diazepam

185. Which of the following statements is NOT true?
    A. in some cases, depression has been associated with low brain norepinephrine levels
    B. brain norepinephrine is metabolized to 3-methoxy-4-hydroxy-phenylglycol (MHPG)
    C. urinary levels of MHPG are statistically lower in groups of seriously depressed patients
    D. desipramine primarily blocks the uptake of norepinephrine
    E. amitriptyline primarily blocks the reuptake of norepinephrine

Questions 186 and 187

A 30-year-old man came to the clinic because over the past two years he has felt constantly edgy, tense, and vigilant. He complains of dizziness, sweating palms, ringing in the ears, and palpitations. These symptoms have been present most of the time and are not limited to discrete periods.

186. The MOST likely axis I diagnosis is
   A. generalized anxiety disorder
   B. panic disorder
   C. obsessive–compulsive disorder
   D. agoraphobia
   E. agoraphobia with panic attacks

187. Anxiety may be a prominent symptom in all of the following EXCEPT
   A. schizophrenic disorder
   B. hypochondriasis
   C. obsessive–compulsive disorder
   D. hyperthyroidism
   E. obsessive–compulsive personality

Questions 188 through 190

A young nursing student was admitted to the hospital for severe headache, nausea, vomiting, stiff neck, and sudden development of a dilated, light-fixed, right pupil. Eyelid ptosis and extraocular muscle weakness were not present. It was later discovered she had put an anticholinergic drug in her eye and that she had a history of multiple hospitalizations for obscure disorders. At one time, she had caused skin abscesses and bacteremia by injecting urine subcutaneously.

She left the hospital against medical advice but was shortly admitted to another hospital with opisthotonos and a history of having been bitten by a sick squirrel.

188. The MOST likely diagnosis is
  A. somatization disorder
  B. malingering
  C. Briquet syndrome
  D. hypochondriasis
  E. factitious disorder with physical symptoms

189. Which of the following statements is NOT true of this disorder?
  A. it is more common in women
  B. family history is not known to be of significance
  C. hospital stay usually ends in discharge against medical advice
  D. patients may assume the identity of a person with great prestige
  E. it may be associated with substance abuse, especially of analgesics

190. Somatization disorder may be differentiated from hypochondriasis in which of the following ways?
  A. there is an earlier age of onset in somatization disorder
  B. there is a more narrow range of somatic symptoms in somatization disorder
  C. somatization disorder is more common in males
  D. there is more association with obsessive–compulsive traits
  E. there is more association with anal traits

Question 191

A 35-year-old woman who has a 15-year history of multiple somatic complaints has been "worked up" and treated by a number of physicians. However, all their efforts have made no impact on her chronic but fluctuating symptoms.

She now complains, in a vague but dramatic manner, of an array of symptoms: nausea, lightheadedness, dyspareunia, irregular menses, shortness of breath, and heartburn. Physical examination and diagnostic testing disclose no abnormalities.

191. The MOST likely diagnosis is
    A. somatization disorder
    B. Münchhausen syndrome
    C. factitious disorder
    D. malingering
    E. hypochondriasis

Questions 192 through 195

A 27-year-old woman, married five years and the mother of two children, comes for an initial outpatient appointment relating a history of "anxiety attacks" characterized by a racing heart, nausea, shortness of breath, trembling, and fear of dying. The attacks began about two months ago, following a minor traffic accident in which she was involved. Since then, she has had 2 to 3 attacks per week. The attacks usually occur at the shopping market, when going out to dinner, or when driving. Although she continues to go out, she now loathes the thought of having to drive and avoids it if at all possible. She relates no precipitating events to the individual attacks and no history of other psychiatric difficulties or depressive symptoms. She describes no other psychosocial stressors.

192. The appropriate axis I diagnosis, using DSM–IV, is
    A. general anxiety disorder with simple phobia (driving a car)
    B. panic disorder with agoraphobia
    C. panic disorder without agoraphobia
    D. panic disorder with agoraphobic tendencies
    E. anxiety disorder, NOS

193. Which of the following would appropriately be listed on DSM–IV, axis IV?
  A. mother of 2 children—twins, age 2
  B. shopping at busy supermarket
  C. minor traffic accident
  D. marriage of 5 years to inattentive husband
  E. all of the above

194. Which of the following might appropriately be considered in the differential diagnosis of this woman?
  A. social phobia
  B. somatization disorder
  C. posttraumatic stress disorder
  D. substance-induced anxiety disorder
  E. all of the above

195. Her axis V diagnosis, current GAF, is
  A. 30
  B. 50
  C. 60
  D. 70
  E. 80

Questions 196 through 199

A 36-year-old white man comes to your office seeking help for a problem that he relates has been plaguing him for some time but that he now wants to "fix" before he gets married. He says that since his late teens (about the time he left home to go to college) he has been pulling the hair from the left side of his head with his left hand. He describes a particular ritual involved: there is a feeling of building tension and desire to pull a strand of hair from his head, with a feeling of relief and relaxation upon completion of the act. Simultaneously, he wishes that he was not engaging in this activity. He has noticeable hair loss on the left side of his head.

He is an accountant and refers you to a copy of an MMPI done several years previously when he saw a psychologist for the same problem. The profile is valid and shows no evidence of psychosis, but endorses several character traits, especially orderliness, rigidity, emotional constriction, obstinacy, and indecisiveness. There is a mild elevation in the depression scale, with other scales being within the norm.

He relates no symptoms of a major affective disorder and, aside from episodic alcohol intoxication, there is no evidence of additional psychopathology.

196. Using DSM–IV, the appropriate axis I diagnosis is
    A. obsessive–compulsive personality disorder
    B. obsessive–compulsive disorder
    C. anxiety disorder, NOS
    D. trichotillomania
    E. psychological factors affecting physical condition

197. An appropriate axis II diagnosis is
    A. obsessive–compulsive personality disorder
    B. obsessive–compulsive disorder
    C. histrionic personality disorder
    D. pervasive developmental disorder
    E. none of the above

198. According DSM–IV, the axis I diagnosis is included under which category?
    A. anxiety disorders
    B. impulse control disorders
    C. dissociative disorders
    D. adjustment disorders
    E. somatoform disorders

199. Trichotillomania is best treated with
    A. anxiolytics with antihistamine properties
    B. imipramine
    C. biofeedback
    D. hypnotherapy
    E. none of the above

Directions (Questions 200 through 203): Each group of questions below consists of lettered headings followed by a list of numbered words,
phrases, or statements. For each numbered word, phrase, or statement,
select the ONE lettered heading that is most closely associated with it.
Each lettered heading may be selected once, more than once, or not at
all.

Match the following personality disorder cluster with the most appro-
priate item. Use each once, more than once, or not at all.
- **A.** cluster A
- **B.** cluster B
- **C.** cluster C

200. Suicide attempts

201. Belief in "the little signal"

202. Alcohol abuse

203. Delightful and infectious laughter

Mental Disorders and DSM–IV

Explanatory Answers

1. (D) PCP is a psychotomimetic drug (like LSD, mescaline, and DMT) that produces a schizophreniform psychosis characterized by hallucinations, paranoia, restlessness, and disturbed thought processes, but with preservation of sensorium. (**Ref. 1,** p. 447)

2. (C) Some patients suffering from depression, as well as personality disorders, schizophrenia, and factitious disorders, may present with descriptive signs and symptoms of memory impairment, slowed speech, behavioral aberrations, and other descriptive qualifiers of dementia. However, if their higher cortical functions remain intact, it is likely they have a pseudodementia due to an axis I, rather than axis III, etiology. (**Ref. 1,** p. 354)

3. (C) If clouding of consciousness is present, as in delirium and intoxication, a diagnosis of amnestic syndrome cannot be made. Amnestic impairment may involve the ability to learn new information or recall previously learned information. (**Ref. 4,** p. 156)

4. (A) Delusional disorder is characterized by the presence of one or more nonbizarre delusions that persist for at least one month. Sensorium remains clear and hallucinations are generally not prominent, although tactile and olfactory hallucinations may be prominent if they are related to the delusional theme. (**Ref. 4,** p. 296)

5. (**E**) Acute cocaine poisoning is most common among intravenous users, but it can also follow "free-basing" (smoking the alkalinized extract). The symptoms are similar to those of acute amphetamine intoxication: elevated blood pressure, hyperthermia, tachycardia, and respiratory depression. (**Ref. 1,** pp. 423–427)

6. (**E**) Serum alcohol levels from 100 to 200 mg/dL are common in patients who have pathological intoxication and form the most secure basis of diagnosis. Clinical signs that are characteristic for ETOH intoxication include slurred speech, unsteady gait, nystagmus, and impairment in attention or memory. (**Ref. 1,** p. 404)

7. (**E**) While there is a syndrome of alcohol-induced sexual dysfunction, this refers to impaired desire, arousal, orgasm, or sexual pain. A paraphilia involves recurrent, intense, sexually arousing fantasies, urges, or behaviors directed towards nonhuman objects or sadomasochistically toward oneself, partner, or children. (**Ref 4,** pp. 195, 522)

8. (**D**) Although delusions may accompany the hallucinosis experienced in alcoholic hallucinations, they are not prominent and usually develop as an explanatory mechanism for the hallucinations. While the hallucinosis typically subsides more rapidly, it may linger for several weeks. (**Ref. 1,** p. 408)

9. (**A**) Brief psychotic disorder involves the sudden onset of positive psychotic symptoms. The essential features of schizophreniform disorder are identical to those of schizophrenia except the total duration of the illness is from 1 to 6 months and impaired social or occupational functioning need not occur. (**Ref. 4,** pp. 290, 302)

10. (**E**) Paraphilias are disorders wherein sexual arousal requires imagery or acts of an unusual nature. Transvestic fetishism, pedophilia, zoophilia, exhibitionism, voyeurism, and sadomasochism fall into this group. All are compulsive and repetitive. Conversion symptoms are classically considered hysterical. (**Ref. 1,** p. 674)

11. **(D)** Anorexia nervosa is primarily a disorder of young women, although about 5% of otherwise typical cases occur in men. Although frequently seen together, anorexia and bulimia represent distinct clinical entities. **(Ref. 1, p. 689)**

12. **(C)** DSM–IV categorization of mood disorders encompasses bipolar disorder, cyclothymia, major depression, dysthymia, and depressive disorder, NOS. Posttraumatic stress disorder is categorized under anxiety disorders. **(Ref. 4, pp. 317, 393)**

13. **(A)** Dysthymic disorder is a chronic, relatively mild condition. It is characterized by at least two years of depressed mood; it has no hypomanic features. **(Ref. 1, p. 556)**

14. **(E)** Approximately 70% to 80% of patients with bipolar affective disorder can be expected to respond in 5 to 14 days at serum lithium levels between 0.8 and 1.2 mEq/L. All other answers regarding bipolar disorder are accurate. **(Ref. 1, p. 553)**

15. **(E)** Uncomplicated bereavement is a normal reaction to the death of a loved one and is not classified as a mental disorder under DSM–IV. A full depressive syndrome may be present with poor appetite, weight loss, and insomnia. However, marked preoccupation with worthlessness, functional impairment, and marked psychomotor retardation are uncommon and suggest that the bereavement is complicated by the development of a major depressive episode. **(Ref. 4, p. 684)**

16. **(D)** The term "melancholia," as used in DSM–IV, is completely descriptive in nature and does not imply any etiology. Another of the diagnostic criteria for a melancholic-type major depression not mentioned is that there is a history of a previous good response to specific and adequate treatment with an antidepressant, such as a tricyclic antidepressant. **(Ref. 4, p. 383)**

17. **(E)** People with major depression superimposed on a dysthymic disorder frequently are referred to as suffering "double depression," and are at greater risk for developing a recurrence of a major depressive episode than those who have a major depressive episode without the occurrence of a concurrent dysthymia. **(Ref. 4, p. 346)**

18. **(A)** The hallmark feature of dysthymia is a chronic disturbance of depressed mood over a two-year time span in which the person is never without depressive symptoms for more than two months. (**Ref. 4,** pp. 345–349)

19. **(D)** If there is no mania, the disorder can not be classified as bipolar. The bipolar I classification refers to the occurrence of a full manic episode. Bipolar II refers to the recurrent major depressive episodes with hypomanic episodes. (**Ref. 4,** p. 350)

20. **(D)** Postconcussional disorder is categorized as a research criteria set under DSM–IV. The essential feature is an acquired impairment in cognitive functioning, accompanied by neurobehavioral derangement—both secondary to a closed head injury. (**Ref. 4,** pp. 703, 704)

21. **(C)** The delusion falls under the category of a thought content disorder. A delusion is a belief, usually false, arrived at by other-than-logical means, that is not subject to change by the normal means of logic and persuasion. It is not a belief ordinarily accepted by other members of the person's culture or religious faith. (**Ref. 1,** p. 278)

22. **(E)** The persistent toxic state brought on by chronic amphetamine-like drug use characterized by paranoia, visual and tactile hallucinations, generalized suspiciousness with ideas of reference, and a clear state of consciousness, is designated amphetamine or similarly acting sympathomimetic-induced psychotic disorder. Early morning awakening is associated with depression. (**Ref. 4,** p. 310)

23. **(E)** Thought insertion is the feeling that thoughts are being planted in one's mind by other people or forces. It is not part of the symptom complex of posttraumatic stress disorder. (**Ref. 4,** p. 424)

24. **(E)** Although one of the symptoms that may occur in posttraumatic stress disorder is a dissociative episode, this is only one symptom of a much larger complex. Posttraumatic stress disorder is classified under the anxiety disorders. Under DSM–IV, multiple personality disorder is now called dissociative identity disorder. (**Ref. 4,** pp. 424, 477)

25. (E) Although personality disorders frequently may predispose an individual to substance abuse or dependence, the concept of dependence refers specifically to an individual's behavioral pattern in which the use of a given drug is given a much higher priority than other behaviors that once had higher value. **(Ref. 1, pp. 384–386)**

26. (D) Factitious disorders are characterized by the deliberate and apparently senseless simulation of physical or mental illness. Conversion, somatization, psychogenic pain disorder, and hypochondriasis are not thought to be under conscious control. **(Ref. 1, p. 632)**

27. (C) If the symptoms are an exacerbation of a preexisting mental disorder, the condition cannot be classified as an adjustment disorder. The stressor may be a single event, or there may be multiple stressors (eg marked financial troubles and marital difficulties). **(Ref. 4, p. 623)**

28. (E) Wernicke's encephalopathy is characterized by ophthalmoplegia and memory loss. In addition, depression, anxiety, disturbance of consciousness, and ataxia may be present. It is produced by a central nervous system deficiency of thiamine. Although beriberi is also a thiamine-deficiency disease, it is characterized by peripheral neuropathy, cardiac hypertrophy, weakness, and edema. **(Ref. 1, p. 359)**

29. (D) Although memory impairment certainly can occur in delirium, it is frequently found in dementia, as well as other syndromes. The hallmark symptom of delirium is an impairment of consciousness, usually seen in association with global impairments of cognitive functions. **(Ref. 1, p. 357)**

30. (C) The only perceptual disturbance listed is a hallucination. Loosening of associations is a disturbance of thought process; delusions are a thought content disorder. **(Ref. 1, p. 341)**

31. (A) Focal neurological signs are uncommon in delirium and, if present, should warrant a specific investigation for a structural lesion. Although autonomic instability is seen frequently in delirium, it is not a neurological sign. **(Ref. 1, p. 343)**

32. (C) Clouding of consciousness is specifically excluded in the diagnostic criteria for amnestic disorder. Clouding of consciousness in the postictal state typically lasts 1 to 2 hours. (**Ref. 1,** pp. 357–359)

33. (E) In general, the body can metabolize approximately one drink per hour. This corresponds to a decrease in the blood alcohol level of approximately 15 to 20 mg/dL per hour. (**Ref. 4,** p. 203)

34. (D) Approximately 25% of suicides are alcoholic, predominantly white males over the age of 35. Alcohol-related disorders also contribute to absenteeism from work, job-related accidents, and low employee productivity. (**Ref. 1,** pp. 803–810; **Ref. 4,** pp. 199–201)

35. (B) The behavior, which is aggressive and atypical for the individual, is usually not remembered and occurs after ingesting an amount of alcohol insufficient to induce intoxication in most people. Because of limited support in the literature for the validity of this condition, it is not included in DSM–IV. (**Ref. 4,** p. 204)

36. (C) Although there may be some transient, mildly delirious features, such as autonomic hyperactivity, transient hallucinations and illusions, and general malaise, the development of a true picture of delirium merits the additional diagnosis of alcohol withdrawal delirium. Alcohol withdrawal may occur after the reduction of heavy and prolonged alcohol use, in addition to cessation. (**Ref. 4,** p. 197)

37. (C) There is no correlation to duration of usage. The essential feature of substance abuse is a maladaptive pattern of substance use manifested by recurrent and significant adverse consequences. (**Ref. 4,** p. 182)

38. (D) Atypical aggressive behavior following minimal alcohol ingestion is typical of what was previously described (DSM–IIIR) as alcohol idiosyncratic intoxication. Although a diagnosis of substance abuse is more likely in individuals who have just started using a substance, some individuals develop a pattern of chronic abuse. (**Ref. 4,** pp. 182, 204)

39. (C) All of the other phobic disorders may be classified as listed. Taphophobia is a specific phobia dealing with the fear of being buried alive. (**Ref. 1,** p. 594; **Ref. 4,** p. 393)

40. (A) Agoraphobia is so infrequently seen in clinical practice without the association of panic attacks that some investigators question its validity as a distinct entity. The core fear of all agoraphobic patients is being placed in a situation where escape or help would not be immediately available in case of sudden incapacitation. (**Ref. 1,** p. 589)

41. (B) Familial expressed emotion is defined as criticism and emotional overinvolvement by family members of schizophrenic patients and is the most consistent powerful predictor of relapse in the nine months following discharge from an inpatient treatment setting. (**Ref. 1,** p. 470)

42. (E) Just as schizophrenia is a pervasive disorder affecting most facets of a patient's life, so must be the treatment intervention. Thus, a combination of medication and psychological and social intervention must be employed to allow for reasonable treatment. Lithium is used in treating bipolar disorder, not schizophrenia. (**Ref. 1,** pp. 481–484)

43. (D) Kernberg believes that the most frequently used pathological defense mechanisms of borderlines are projective identification and splitting. The "mirror transference" is one of the specific types of transference Kohut has described as arising in the treatment of a narcissistic personality. (**Ref. 1,** pp. 739–740)

44. (A) Mood-incongruent delusions are much less likely to be found in major depression than are mood-congruent delusions and should alert the clinician to the possibility of a schizophrenic disorder. In general, delusions do not dominate the clinical picture of a mood disorder. (**Ref. 4,** p. 377)

45. (A) If the bereaved person is preoccupied with guilt and worthlessness or shows marked psychomotor retardation, a major depressive disorder would be suspected. The diagnosis of major depressive disorder is generally not given unless the symptoms are still present two months after the loss. (**Ref. 4,** p. 684)

46. (D) The diagnosis of adjustment disorder should not be made if the condition represents an exacerbation of another mental disorder. The symptoms must develop within three months of the onset of the stressor. (**Ref. 4,** p. 623)

47. (B) Although some premorbidly obese patients may lose up to 25% of their body weight, the descriptive criteria is a body weight 15% below that expected. The term "anorexia" is a misnomer because loss of appetite is rare. (**Ref. 4,** p. 539)

48. (D) Somatic hallucinations are indicative of other mental disorders. Somatic hallucinations are also known as cenesthetic hallucinations. (**Ref. 4,** pp. 462–465)

49. (C) A high IQ and the development of meaningful language in the age range of 5 to 7 years are important prognostic indicators in infantile autism. Adult outcome studies indicate that about two-thirds of autistic adults remain severely handicapped. (**Ref. 1,** p. 1058)

50. (E) The hallucinations accompanying alcohol withdrawal delirium are most frequently either visual or tactile, but they also may be auditory. Serum ammonia levels are not etiologically associated with alcohol withdrawal delirium. This syndrome is also known as delirium tremens. (**Ref. 4,** pp. 129–131)

51. (E) A state of clouded consciousness is the essential feature of delirium. The term "clouded consciousness" refers to a reduction in the clarity of awareness of the environment and self. Hallucinations are not included. (**Ref. 1,** p. 338)

52. (A) Cocaine is a psychostimulant that produces a marked sense of exhilaration, self-confidence, and euphoria. As the stimulus wears off, however, the user feels dysphoric, fatigued, and somnolent, although the patient may be unable to sleep due to agitation. Formicative hallucinations are the feeling of bugs or vermin crawling under the skin and are commonly associated with cocaine or amphetamine psychosis. Pupillary dilatation occurs with acute cocaine intoxication. (**Ref. 1,** pp. 423–427)

53. (E) Dementia may be caused by a plethora of conditions. It is vital to diagnose early and treat those conditions that are reversible, such as hyperthyroidism, vitamin deficiency, heavy metal poisoning, and normal pressure hydrocephalus. Depression may mimic dementia symptoms, but, in fact, it is considered a pseudodementia. Amyloid-B is associated with Alzheimer's disease. **(Ref. 1,** pp. 345–346)

54. (A) The Klein–Levin syndrome is a rare disease most common in adolescent males, and it is thought to be due to intermittent dysfunction in the limbic or hypothalamic areas of the brain. The major symptoms are periodic hypersomnia and excessive eating. Behavioral abnormalities such as sexual disinhibition or hyperactivity, preference for sweets, some degree of amnesia, depression, and insomnia following the attack occur in conjunction. **(Ref. 1,** p. 711)

55. (C) During the active phase of psychosis, to meet the criteria for schizophrenia, two of the following must be present simultaneously: delusions, prominent hallucinations, incoherence or marked loosening of associations, catatonic behavior, flat or grossly inappropriate affect. Although marked social isolation or withdrawal is seen frequently with schizophrenic patients, it is a characteristic associated with the prodromal or residual phases and does not enter into the diagnosis during the active phases of psychosis. **(Ref. 4,** pp. 275–285)

56. (A) DSM–IV is a categorical classification that divides mental disorders into types based on criteria sets with defining features. A categorical approach to classification works best when all members of a diagnostic class are homogeneous, when there are clear boundaries between classes, and when the different classes are mutually exclusive. **(Ref. 4,** p. xxii)

57. (C) The essential feature of a dementia is the development of multiple cognitive deficits that include memory impairment and at least one of the following cognitive disturbances: aphasia, apraxia, agnosia, or a disturbance in executive functioning. These may be accompanied by delirium, delusions, or depressed mood. There is no qualifier for hallucinations under DSM–IV. **(Ref. 4,** pp. 133–143)

58. (B) Compared with the general population, first-degree biological relatives of individuals with dementia of the Alzheimer's type (early onset) are more likely to develop the disorder. Late-onset cases may also have a genetic component. (**Ref. 4,** p. 142)

59. (C) Giggling may accompany cannabis intoxication but is not typically associated with alcohol intoxication. All of the other symptoms listed are consistent with alcohol intoxication. (**Ref. 4,** pp. 197, 217)

60. (D) In dementia, there is global cognitive impairment without clouding of consciousness. The patient's personality is also affected in dementia. (**Ref. 1,** p. 345)

61. (C) A fluctuating level of consciousness is a major diagnostic criterion for delirium and an exclusion criterion for other organic syndromes. Some have suggested that the inability of delirious patients to maintain attention is the central feature of delirium. (**Ref. 1,** p. 341)

62. (E) No single symptom is pathognomonic of schizophrenia— the diagnosis involves the recognition of a constellation of signs and symptoms. Characteristic symptoms include delusions, hallucinations, disorganized speech, grossly disorganized or catatonic behavior, and "negative" symptoms (affective flattening, avolition). (**Ref. 4,** pp. 274–285)

63. (G) Cocaine intoxication typically causes elation, euphoria, heightened self-esteem, gregariousness, hypervigilance, and stereotyped behavior. This "high" may quickly progress to paranoia, anger, delusional grandiosity, impulsivity, and aggression. Frequently cocaine intoxication mimics a manic state. (**Ref. 4,** p. 223)

64. (A) Individuals with amnestic disorder are impaired in their ability to learn new information or are unable to recall previously learned information or events. The ability to learn and recall new information is by definition always affected. (**Ref. 4,** p. 156)

65. (F) Some patients taking reserpine develop a major depressive episode to the point of becoming suicidal. This is not particularly infrequent. (**Ref. 1,** pp. 570–571)

66. (B) The essential feature of Rett's disorder is the development of multiple specific deficits following a period of normal functioning after birth. It is typically associated with severe or profound mental retardation. (**Ref. 4,** p. 71)

67. (F) In addition to reserpine, methyldopa is another antihypertensive that may cause a depressive syndrome. Of the beta blockers, propranolol is the best known for causing depression. (**Ref. 1,** pp. 570–571)

68. (E) "Positive" symptoms of schizophrenia include hallucinations, delusions, disorganized speech, and grossly disorganized or catatonic behavior. "Negative" symptoms include restrictions in the range and intensity of emotional expression (affective flattening), alogia (deficit in the fluency and productivity of thought and speech), and avolition. (**Ref. 4,** pp. 274–275)

69. (B) "Alcohol hallucinations" is a term for hallucinations occurring during alcohol withdrawal that is not used in DSM–IV. Under DSM–IV, it would be termed alcohol-induced psychotic disorder (with hallucinations) with onset during withdrawal. The most common hallucinations are auditory. (**Ref. 1,** p. 408)

70. (D) The essential features of primary degenerative dementia are an insidious onset and a gradual course. Of all patients with dementia, 50% to 60% have dementia of the Alzheimer's type. (**Ref. 1,** pp. 349–350)

71. (A) Multi-infarct dementia is characterized by a stepwise, deteriorating course, with a patchy distribution of defects, and by focal neurological signs and symptoms. There tends to be a greater preservation of personality in patients with vascular dementia. (**Ref. 1,** p. 353)

72. (B) The transsexual, unlike the transvestite, is uncomfortable with his/her anatomic sex. While the term transsexualism is popular in the literature and was used in DSM–IIIR, under DSM–IV the correct terminology for this disorder is gender identity disorder. (**Ref. 1,** p. 682)

73. (**A**)   Sexual activity may involve the fetishism object alone, such as male masturbation into a woman's shoe. The particular fetish is linked to someone closely involved with the patient during childhood and has some quality associated with that loved, needed, or even traumatizing person. (**Ref. 1,** p. 676)

74. (**C**)   The transvestite cross-dresses for sexual excitement, not because he or she wishes to be the opposite sex. Transvestic fetishism typically begins in childhood or early adolescence. (**Ref. 1,** p. 677)

75. (**B**)   Somatization disorder is also called Briquet's syndrome. The disorder is chronic, with symptoms present for several years and beginning before age 30. (**Ref. 4,** pp. 446–450)

76. (**A**)   The diagnosis of conversion disorder is unique in DSM–IV in that it depends on the determination of etiology; psychological factors must be judged to be causative. (**Ref. 4,** pp. 452–457)

77. (**C**)   One of the diagnostic criteria for somatoform pain disorder is that there is only one major symptom—pain. This factor helps in differentiating it from other conditions such as somatization disorder and hypochondriasis. (**Ref. 4,** p. 458)

78. (**A**)   Separation anxiety disorder is excessive anxiety, for at least four weeks, concerning separation from those to whom the child is attached. Onset of the disorder is before age 18. When not with a major attachment figure, children with this disorder may exhibit recurrent instances of social withdrawal, apathy, sadness, or difficulty concentrating on work or play. (**Ref. 1,** pp. 1104–1105)

79. (**B**)   In some cases of major depression, especially in boys, conduct disturbances or full disorders may occur within the context of a major depressive episode and resolve with the resolution of the depressive episode. (**Ref. 1,** p. 1116)

80. **(C)** This is a very important differential diagnosis. The pseudo-dementia associated with depression is usually totally reversible. (**Ref. 1,** p. 354)

81. **(B)** The essential feature of cyclothymia is a chronic mood disturbance of at least two years' duration (one year for children and adolescents), involving numerous hypomanic episodes and numerous periods of mild depression insufficient to meet criteria for major depression. Also, the patient is without euthymia for more than two months. (**Ref. 4,** p. 363)

82. **(A)** In dysthymic disorder, there is no hypomania. In adults, there must be a chronically depressed mood that occurs for most of the day, more days than not, for at least two years. (**Ref. 4,** p. 345)

83. **(A)** In substance abuse disorders, duration is a major diagnostic criterion, as a pattern of maladaptive behavior is integral to the diagnosis. The person may continue to use the substance, despite a history of undesirable consequences. (**Ref. 4,** p. 182)

84. **(B)** In panic disorder, one or more attacks have been followed by a period of at least a month of persistent fear of having an attack. Typically, there are recurrent panic attacks several times a week or even daily. (**Ref. 4,** p. 397)

85. **(C)** The essential features of schizophrenia and schizophreniform disorder are the same, with the exception that their duration, including prodromal, active, and residual phases, is less than six months in schizophreniform disorder. (**Ref. 4,** p. 274)

86. **(B)** The essential feature of delusional disorder is the presence of one or more non-bizarre delusions that persist for at least one month. Subtypes, based upon the delusional theme, include erotomanic, grandiose, jealous, persecutory, and somatic. (**Ref. 4,** p. 296)

87. **(E)** For the diagnosis of major depressive episode, an individual must experience either depressed mood or loss of interest or pleasure in almost all activities with associated symptoms for a period of at least two weeks. Failure to have the disorder for at least two

weeks would result in the diagnosis of a depressive disorder, not otherwise specified. (**Ref. 4,** p. 320)

88. (F) Posttraumatic stress disorder (PTSD) can begin any time after the occurrence of the stressor, but the full syndrome usually does not evolve immediately. When the onset of symptoms is at least six months after the trauma, the diagnosis is delayed onset. (**Ref. 4,** p. 424)

89. (B) Patients with agoraphobia generally are thrown into a state of extreme anxiety when placed in a situation in which they fear they would be helpless were they to be incapacitated. Both open places and public places eg, crowded stores, public transportation, and elevators pose a threat to such patients. (**Ref. 4,** p. 396)

90. (C) The essential feature of social phobia is fear of exposure to the scrutiny of others and of behaving in a humiliating or embarrassing fashion. The response may take the form of a situationally bound or predisposed panic attack. (**Ref. 4,** p. 411)

91. (B) The essential features of attention-deficit hyperactivity disorder are developmentally inappropriate inattention, impulsivity, and hyperactivity. Symptoms that cause impairment must have been present before age 7. (**Ref. 4,** p. 78)

92. (A) The essential feature of conduct disorder is violation of the rights of others or of age-appropriate societal norms. The behaviors fall into four main groupings: aggressive conduct, nonaggressive conduct, deceitfulness or theft, and serious violation of rules. (**Ref. 4,** p. 85)

93. (C) The essential feature of selective mutism is persistent refusal to talk in one or more major social situations. Children with this disorder generally have normal language skills, though some have delayed language development and abnormalities of articulation. (**Ref. 4,** p. 114)

94. (D) The essential feature in oppositional–defiant disorder, as the name suggests, is disobedient, negativistic, and provocative behavior toward authority figures. Behaviors that typically occur are losing temper, arguing with adults, active defiance, deliberately annoying others, blaming others, and being spiteful and vindictive. (**Ref. 4,** p. 91)

95. (**E**)   Pervasive developmental disorder, not otherwise specified, should be used when there is a qualitative impairment in the development of reciprocal social interaction and verbal and nonverbal communication skills; however, the criteria are not meant for autistic disorder, schizophrenia, Rett's disorder, Asperger's disorder, or childhood disintegrative disorder. (**Ref. 4,** p. 77)

96. (**F**)   Infantile autism is more accurately termed autistic disorder under DSM–IV. The essential features of this disorder constitute a severe form of pervasive developmental disorder, with onset by 36 months. The features involve qualitative impairment in reciprocal social interaction, verbal and nonverbal communication, and imaginative activity, and a markedly restricted repertoire of activities and interest. (**Ref. 4,** p. 66)

97. (**D**)   Sleep terror (parvor nocturnus) is an arousal in the first third of the night from deep non-REM sleep (stage III or IV), almost invariably heralded by a piercing scream, and accompanied by behavioral manifestations of intense anxiety bordering on panic. The individual experiencing the sleep terror has minimal, if any, recall of the event itself. (**Ref. 1,** p. 711)

98. (**D**)   Sleepwalking (somnambulism) occurs usually during the first third of the night in deep non-REM sleep (stages III or IV), is accompanied by an absence of dreaming, does not always progress to walking, and is characterized by semi-purposeful automatism and morning amnesia on the part of the patient. (**Ref. 1,** p. 712)

99. (**A**)   A nightmare (dream anxiety attack) is an awakening from REM sleep usually later in the nocturnal sleep cycle, with vivid recall of an extended and disturbing dream, accompanied by anxiety and some autonomic arousal. (**Ref. 1,** p. 711)

100. (**E**)   In most cases, functional enuresis occurs during non-REM sleep. In a few cases, it occurs during REM sleep. When occurring during REM sleep, the child may recall a dream involving urination or water. (**Ref. 1,** p. 1102)

101. (C) Sleep-related bruxism (teeth grinding) occurs primarily in non-REM sleep, most prominently in stage two, and consists of rhythmic masseter muscle activity in sleep. In 5% to 10% of the population, it is severe enough to cause tooth damage. **(Ref. 1, p. 713)**

102. (A) Nocturnal penile tumescence occurs in all healthy males, mainly during REM sleep. Nocturnal penile tumescence monitoring is currently used to distinguish organic from psychogenic causes of impotency. **(Ref. 1, p. 701)**

103. (A), 104. (A), 105. (B), 106. (B) Reduction of clarity of awareness of environment (clouding of consciousness) is characteristic of delirium, in contrast to dementia in which awareness and alertness are presented in the early stages of the illness and become impaired late in the illness. Misperceptions in the form of illusions, or hallucinations (visual) are more common in delirium and less frequent in dementia. Dementia has a chronic course, which may last for months or years. The course for delirium may be hours or days. Alzheimer-type is the most common dementia. Histopathologically, Alzheimer's primary degenerative dementia seems the same in both the senile and presenile forms. The histopathology characteristics of Alzheimer's disease are senile plaques and neurofibrillary tangles. **(Ref. 1,** pp. 343, 612–615, 624–626; **Ref. 3,** pp. 101, 106, 107)

107. (A), 108. (B), 109. (A), 110. (B), 111 (A) Disorders in thought process (form) differ from disorders of thought content in that the former refer to the way thoughts are connected or associated. In normal thinking, the thoughts are logical, sequential, and goal-directed. Thought content answers the question "What is the thought?" In circumstantiality, unnecessary elaborate detail is given, but eventually the point is reached. Delusions are fixed, false beliefs from which the person cannot be dissuaded. In word salad, the words have no logical, coherent connection. Obsessions are disturbing, intrusive, and persistent thoughts. Neologisms are words made up by and understood by the patient. **(Ref. 1,** pp. 277–278; **Ref. 3,** pp. 28–30)

112. **(A)** Delusions typically are not a part of the paranoid personality disorder. If delusion is present, another disorder (such as delusional disorder or paranoid schizophrenia) should be considered. (**Ref. 3,** pp. 183–184; **Ref. 4,** pp. 634–636)

113. **(E)** Schizotypal personalities may be distinguished from those with schizophrenia by the absence of psychosis in the former. Originally, the delusion of thought insertion was one of the primary diagnosis criteria Schneider described for schizophrenia. (**Ref. 2,** pp. 1369– 1370)

114. **(C)** The diagnosis of passive-aggressive personality is reserved for diagnosis in adulthood. Similar patterns of resistance and opposition in children are diagnosed as oppositional defiant disorder. (**Ref. 3,** pp. 191–192; **Ref. 4,** pp. 733–734)

115. **(A)** Preoccupation with details is characteristic of obsessive–compulsive disorder. Persons with dependent personality disorder tend to subordinate their own needs to those of others and get others to assume responsibility for important areas in their lives. They lack self-confidence and may be intensely uncomfortable when alone for brief periods. Dependent personality disorder is prevalent approximately three times as often in women as in men. (**Ref. 2,** p. 1380)

116. **(B)** Mental retardation is listed on axis II according to DSM–IV. Disorders usually diagnosed in childhood or adolescence, such as disorders in reading, mathematics, written expression, and learning disorders, NOS, are listed on axis I. (**Ref. 1,** p. 315; **Ref. 4,** p. 26)

117. **(A)** Rigidity of behavioral patterns and blaming others for one's problems are characteristic of all personality disorders. Hypersensitivity to criticism and chronic suspiciousness suggest a paranoid personality disorder. (**Ref. 3,** pp. 183–184, 192)

118. **(D)** According to the 1948 Kinsey study, 10% of males are homosexual. Subsequent studies, however, indicate a lower percent. According to the U.S. Bureau of Census (1988), the male prevalence rate for homosexuality is 2 to 3%. Other studies suggest even lower rates. (**Ref. 1,** p. 658)

119. (B) Homosexuality was seen not as a pathological disorder but rather as an alternative lifestyle by the American Psychiatric Association in 1973. This was reflected in its exclusion from the DSM–III and DSM–IIIR. Recognition, though, had been given to ego-dysfunction homosexuality in the DSM–III. This is no longer included in DSM–IV. (**Ref. 1,** pp. 658, 662; **Ref. 4,** p. 493)

120. (C) Dyspareunia is considered to be much more common in women than in men. The incidence of dyspareunia is unknown. (**Ref. 1,** p. 666; Ref. 4, pp. 511–513)

121. (C) Approximately 35% to 40% of men seeking help for sexual disorders have premature ejaculation as a major complaint. It is felt that this problem is more common among college-educated men. However, the true incidence of this disorder is not known. (**Ref. 1,** p. 666)

122. (A) The schizotypal personality disorder is characterized by a pervasive pattern of peculiarities of ideation, appearance, behavior, and deficits in interpersonal relationships. (**Ref. 4,** pp. 641–645)

123. (D) A grandiose sense of self-importance may occur in the person with antisocial personality disorder; however, it is an associated feature rather than diagnostic. A grandiose sense of self-importance is a core feature of the narcissistic personality disorder. (**Ref. 4,** pp. 644–647)

124. (E) The deficits of word recognition skills and reading comprehension may not be explainable by mental retardation, inadequate school, or visual or hearing defect. There also may not be a specific identifiable neurologic disorder producing the deficits. This disorder frequently is associated with attention-deficit hyperactivity disorder but is not caused by it. (**Ref. 4,** pp. 49, 50)

125. (B) Cluster A personality disorders are more common in a biological relative of a schizophrenic patient than in controls. This group of disorders tends to use projection and fantasy as frequent defense mechanisms. (**Ref. 1,** pp. 731, 733–734; **Ref. 4,** pp. 629–630)

126. (A) This group of personality disorders tends to use dissociations, acting out, splitting, neurotic denial, and devaluation as frequently relied upon defense mechanisms. (**Ref. 1,** pp. 731, 733–734; **Ref. 4,** pp. 629–630)

127. (C) Patients with a personality disorder falling within this group tend to use isolation, passive aggression, and hypochondriasis as defense mechanisms. (**Ref. 1,** pp. 731, 733–734; **Ref. 4,** pp. 629–630)

128. (A) The persons with schizoid personality disorders have a life-long pattern of social withdrawal. Their affect is constricted and they may appear indifferent, cold, and aloof. They may seem indifferent to the approval of others. (**Ref. 1,** pp. 735–736; **Ref. 4,** p. 629)

129. (B) Cognitive and perceptual disorders (oddities of thought, perception, and speech) are characteristics of individuals with schizotypal personality disorder. (**Ref. 1,** pp. 736–737; **Ref. 4,** p. 629)

130. (E) The histrionic patient uses emotional display both to obtain attention and desired goals and to evade unwanted external responsibilities and unpleasant inner affects. Thus, the external emotional display and excess are coupled with an internal shallowness. There often is a disturbed ability to maintain deep, long-lasting attachments. (**Ref. 1,** pp. 741–742; **Ref. 4,** p. 629)

131. (C) The narcissistic personality disorder tends to have interpersonal relationships characterized by envy and idealization or by devaluation and manipulation. This is secondary to the grandiose sense of self-importance, which is a core feature of the narcissist. (**Ref. 1,** pp. 742–743; **Ref. 4,** p. 629)

132. (D) Persons with borderline personality disorder show irritability in many areas of functioning, including a persistently unstable sense of self and unstable and intense interpersonal relationships (eg substance abuse, suicidal behavior, inappropriate anger, and affective instability). (**Ref. 1,** pp. 739–741; **Ref. 4,** p. 629)

133. (F) Hypersensitivity to negative evaluation is the central feature of avoidant personality disorder. This leads to social isolation, inhibition, and withdrawal from social involvement. (**Ref. 1,** pp. 743–744; **Ref. 4,** p. 629)

134. (C) Persons with a borderline personality disorder are intolerant of being alone. Their sense of well-being is dependent on having other people with them. Fear of abandonment, rejection, and loss of external structure or a "holding" relationship lead to feelings of panic. (**Ref. 4,** pp. 650–654)

135. (B) It was hypothesized that during the rapprochement subphase of development, the child's efforts to separate and gain autonomy from its mother were resisted by responses that were punitive or engendered severe separation fears. (**Ref. 2,** p. 1389)

136. (D) Defense mechanisms characteristic of an obsessive–compulsive personality disorder are isolation, reaction formation, and displacement. A higher functioning obsessive–compulsive will no doubt use a fair amount of sublimation. Splitting is a quite primitive defense mechanism whereby external objects are experienced as either "all good" or "all bad." It is not characteristic of obsessive–compulsive personality disorders. (**Ref. 1,** pp. 746–747; **Ref. 4,** pp. 733–734)

137. (C) The defense mechanisms described by Freud as central to the obsessive–compulsive personality are isolation, undoing, and reaction formation. (**Ref. 1,** p. 600)

138. (A) The passive–aggressive personality disorder (called negativistic personality disorder in DSM–IV) usually lacks assertiveness and is unstable to express needs and feelings directly. Verbal threats, though not always appropriate, are direct and would therefore not likely be used by such persons. (**Ref. 1,** pp. 746, 747)

139. (B) Persons with narcissistic personality disorder have little capacity for empathy or sympathy. Their involvement with others is based on what they can get out of it, that is, exploit from it. The person with an avoidant personality disorder sees himself as socially inept. The person with borderline personality disorder has a poor sense of self-identity and unstable image of self. Preoccupation with detail is characteristic of the obsessive–compulsive personality disorder. (**Ref. 1,** pp. 739–745)

140. (**C**)   Sporadic is not described as a type of memory disturbance seen in dissociative amnesia. In localized amnesia, there is failure to recall all events from a certain period of time. In systematized amnesia, there is a loss of memory for certain categories of information. In selective amnesia, a person can recall some, but not all, events in a specific time period. In continuous amnesia, there is a failure to recall all events at and after (to current time) events. (**Ref. 4,** p. 478)

141. (**B**)   Dissociative fugue is almost always limited to a single episode. In dissociative identity disorder, there are repeated shifts of identity occurring over time. In dissociative fugue, there is sudden unexpected travel away from home with the associated assumption of a new identity and an inability to recall one's previous identity. Following recovery, there is no recollection of events that took place during the fugue. (**Ref. 4,** pp. 481–487)

142. (**A**)   According to DSM–IV, the essential feature of the dissociative disorders is a disruption in the integrated function of consciousness, memory, identity, or perception of the environment. (**Ref. 4,** p. 477)

143. (**A**)   Patterns of perceiving and thinking are distinct and consistent for each personality state. Each personality is felt to separate and behave as a unitary or single being. Behavior or attitudes are determined by that personality when it is dominant. The personalities may have separate names. (**Ref. 1,** pp. 644–645)

144. (**E**)   Lack of support from significant others during childhood has been identified as one of the contributing factors to the development of the dissociative identity disorder. Answer A—approximately 5% of all psychiatric patients are believed to have this disorder. Answer B—the disorder most commonly occurs in late adolescence and young adulthood. Answer C—several studies have indicated that the disorder occurs more frequently in first-degree biological relatives than in the general population. Answer D—while it is true that most people with the disorder are women,

the percent diagnosed count is higher—90% to 100%. It is felt that the number of men having the diagnosis is underreported and that many of the men enter the criminal justice system. (**Ref. 1,** pp. 644–645)

145. (D) Somnambulism (or sleepwalking) is not categorized as a dissociative disorder. It is included as a parasomnia sleep disorder type. It is similar to the dissociative fugue disorder, which typically begins not in sleep but when the person is awake. Parasomnia is a disorder characterized by abnormal behavioral or a psychological event occurring in association with sleep stages or sleep–wake transition. (**Ref. 4,** pp. 579, 587–591)

146. (D) Although persons with anorexia nervosa may exercise for hours to avoid weight gain, this is not one of the diagnostic criteria. (**Ref. 4,** pp. 539–545)

147. (E) Amenorrhea is not required for a diagnosis of bulimia; however, it is needed to diagnose anorexia nervosa. In binge eating, a large amount of food is consumed during a discrete period of time. The individual feels out of control during the episode. For a diagnosis of bulimia, these episodes must occur a minimum of twice per week over a three-month period. In order to prevent weight gain, compensating behavior such as fasting and the misuse of diuretics takes place. (**Ref. 4,** pp. 545–550)

148. (B) Most bulimic patients maintain their interest in sexual activeness. Anorexic patients tend to lose interest in sexual matters. (**Ref. 1,** p. 696)

149. (E) Tics are involuntary, rapid, repetitive, nonrhythmic motion movements or vocalizations. Although they may be exacerbated in response to stress, they do not serve the purpose of neutralizing anxiety or the stereotypic movement in compulsions, nor do they have the intentional aspect as seen in stereotypic movement disorder. They are experienced as irresistible but can be suppressed for different periods of time. During periods of focused attention or sleep, tics will be decreased. (**Ref. 1,** pp. 1080–1087)

150. (C) The occurrence of Tourette's syndrome in members of the same family supports the view that this and other tic disorders are part of a genetic vulnerability. There is evidence that in some families Tourette's is transmitted in an autosomal dominant fashion. (**Ref. 1,** p. 1080; **Ref. 4,** pp. 102–103)

151. (D) The mean age for the onset for bipolar I disorder is 30. Age of onset ranges from childhood (age 5) to 50 years and older in rare cases. Bipolar I disorder has a prevalence that is equal for men and women and from race to race. The incidence of bipolar I disorder does appear higher in the upper socioeconomic group, possibly because of biased diagnostic practices. A strong genetic component is believed to be present in bipolar I disorder. Family, adoption, and twin studies have all supported this. Linkage studies supporting a genetic component show hope for definitive evidence. However, at this time, no genetic association has been consistently replicated in the linkage studies. (**Ref. 1,** pp. 517–522; **Ref. 4,** pp. 350–358)

152. (B) In a follow-up study at four years of persons with bipolar disorder, all items were found to be of poor outcome except being female. On the particular study, being male puts a person at risk for a poor outcome. (**Ref. 1,** p. 539)

153. (C) Marked impairment in normal functioning is not seen in hypomania but rather in mania. Its presence or the presence of psychotic symptoms differentiate the more serious mania from hypomania. All the other items (A, B, D, and E) are seen in both mania and hypomania. (**Ref. 2,** pp. 211–212)

154. (A) Although delusions may well occur as part of a manic episode, they are not part of the DSM–IV descriptive criteria. A DSM–IV restriction is that at no time during the disturbance have there been delusions or hallucinations for as long as two weeks in the absence of prominent mood symptoms. The typical delusions, when they occur, are consistent with the patient's mood, and tend to be a development of grandiose ideas. (**Ref. 3,** pp. 211–212; **Ref. 4,** p. 332)

155. (D) Activity during a manic episode tends to be characterized by excess and chaos. Although at times there may be a superficial appearance of compulsiveness, if viewed in a more in-depth, longitudinal fashion, this will be seen to be quite disorganized. The etiology of "maniacal strength" is unclear, but it has certainly been documented. (**Ref. 4,** p. 328–329)

156. (C) In Beck's comprehensive, structured theory of depression, a cognitive triad consisting of negative cognitions regarding oneself, the world, and one's future is considered. Interpersonal relationships are not specifically addressed as an individual category. Items A, B, D, and E are all contained within this triad. (**Ref. 1,** p. 860)

157. (A) In depression, one's orientation to person, place, and time is intact. Disorientation is considered a symptom of an organic brain disorder. In depression in the elderly, some signs of a dementia may appear; this condition is referred to as a pseudodementia. In severe depression, delusions do develop. These may have guilt, sinfulness, worthlessness, etc., included in the content. Failure to care for one's personal hygiene is seen in depression as behavior becomes more regressive. Thought blocking usually connected with schizophrenia disorder is also seen in severe depression. As part of their negative view of the world and themselves, depressed individuals will overemphasize the bad in their lives. In their countertransference to these patients, it is important that the therapist still be able to identify and understand the distortion and not accept it as the full story. (**Ref. 1,** pp. 536–537)

158. (A) Disorganized speech is more likely to be seen in catatonic or disorganized schizophrenia. Persons with paranoid schizophrenia are more likely to be older at the onset of their illness and have been able to develop themselves socially and psychologically, having more resources available to them to help them through their illness. (**Ref. 1,** pp. 470–471)

159. (B) Thought blocking is seen in severe depression and schizophrenia. It is reflected in an abrupt cessation of speech before the topic of conversation is completed. The delay that follows may be prolonged. Abrupt changes (not cessations) before the topic of discussion is completed may be seen in mania, but this is more likely due to flight of ideas or disorganization of ideas. (**Ref. 1,** p. 475; **Ref. 2,** p. 29; **Ref. 4,** pp. 328–329)

160. (C) The "four As" of Eugen Bleuler (1911) are autism, associations, affect, and ambivalence. Bleuler felt that the four were fundamental symptoms of the illness. He believed that hallucinations and delusions were often associated with schizophrenia but were secondary and not essential to the diagnosis. **(Ref. 2,** p. 143)

161. (A) Delusions of infidelity (delusional jealousy) are false beliefs, arrived at by other-than-logical means, derived from pathological jealousy that one's lover is unfaithful. It is unlikely that schizophrenics would be able to maintain an intimate interpersonal relationship of sufficient intensity for them to believe that they have an unfaithful lover. In general, erotic delusions are unusual in schizophrenics. The other types of delusions listed are quite frequently seen in schizophrenia. **(Ref. 1,** pp. 470–475)

162. (D) Under DSM–IV, the subtypes of schizophrenia include paranoid, catatonic, disorganized, undifferentiated, and residual. The diagnosis of a particular subtype may change over time and is determined by the clinical picture of a current episode of the illness. Simple schizophrenia is now called simple deteriorative disorder and is listed in DSM–IV "Criteria Sets and Axes Provided for Further Study." Research criteria include the progressive development over a year in functions, deepening of negative symptoms, and problems in socialization. **(Ref. 2,** p. 145; **Ref. 4,** pp. 278–290, 713–714)

163. (D) The positive symptoms of schizophrenia are also referred to as florid, productive, or type I symptoms, and include delusions, hallucinations, and bizarre or agitated behavior. They are associated with an acute onset, a history of exacerbations and remissions, normal premorbid functioning, and a favorable response to antipsychotic medication. Negative symptoms such as apathy are associated with poor outcome and poor response to treatment. **(Ref. 1,** p. 474)

164. (D) Thought blocking, a disorder in thought processing, is likely to be seen in the illness itself. The other items, however, may be seen weeks or even months before the illness of schizophrenia is fully expressed. **(Ref. 1,** pp. 476–478)

165. (C) There are two major ocular abnormalities in schizophrenia: unusually frequent blinking and abnormal rapid eye movements. The abnormal rapid eye movements (saccades) during attempts to follow a moving object smoothly are seen in approximately 50% to 80% of patients. (**Ref. 1,** p. 478; **Ref. 2,** p. 162)

166. (C) Suicide may be precipitated by a desire to escape the mental torture, feelings of emptiness and depression, or hallucinated commands. Particular risk factors include a young age, being early in the course of the illness, a college education with high ambitions, a fluctuating course of exacerbations and remissions, and expressed feelings of depression and hopelessness. People who have chronic symptomatology (who are advanced in the course of their illness) tend to be less likely to try to take their lives. (**Ref. 1,** p. 462; **Ref. 4,** p. 280)

167. (D) Aprosodia is an inability to understand or create the usual emotional inflections of speech. It is not infrequent to see this in a schizophrenic patient. (**Ref. 1,** p. 478)

168. (A) For the diagnosis of schizophrenia, according to DSM–IV, there must be continuous signs of the disturbance for at least six months, including an active phase of at least one week. This is, of course, unless the symptoms have been successfully treated. (**Ref. 4,** p. 285)

169. (D) The term "residual" describes a subtype of schizophrenia and is not used to describe the course of the disorder. All the other terms (A, B, C, E) are used in DSM–IV to describe the longitudinal course. (**Ref. 1,** pp. 286–290)

170. (A) The loss of intellectual abilities, memory impairment, "constructional difficulties," personality change, and a clear state of consciousness are indicative of a dementia. Since he is 55, this patient has a "dementia of the Alzheimer's type with early onset." From the history, physical examination, and laboratory tests, there is nothing to indicate any axis III disorder. (**Ref. 4,** pp. 139)

171. (E) Given the data available, no diagnosis can be given on axis II. An investigation of Mr. Jones's lifelong relationship with others and patterns of defense mechanisms would be required before considering an axis II diagnosis. (**Ref. 2,** pp. 176–179)

172. **(C)** Chorea and other movement deficits are more likely to be seen in the subcortical dementias, such as Huntington's disease and Parkinson's disease. (**Ref. 1,** pp. 349, 1159)

173. **(B)** The GAF would be approximately 35. The man is showing major impairment in several areas. He is unable to manage his day-to-day activities, becomes disoriented to places, and shows deterioration in his intellectual functions. His disheveled appearance suggests early impairment in maintaining personal hygiene. (**Ref. 4,** p. 12)

174. **(C)** Alzheimer's disease, a cortical dementia, is the most common cause of presenile dementia. Pick's disease, also a cortical dementia, is rare compared to Alzheimer's. Tertiary syphilis and myxedema would have been detected in the appropriate laboratory studies. Normal pressure hydrocephalus is an example of a subcortical dementia with a classical triad of symptoms: dementia, ataxia, and urinary incontinence. (**Ref. 3,** pp. 114–120)

175. **(C)** Major depression (single episode) is the most likely axis I diagnosis. The woman's three-month history of physical complaints without demonstrated physiopathology, sleep disturbance, weight loss, anhedonia, and lack of any previous psychiatric problems strongly suggests major depression as a diagnosis. Lack of any previous psychiatric diagnosis in a 40-year-old woman, as well as no history of manic periods, rules against bipolar or schizoaffective disorder. Hypochondriasis is a consideration here; however, the symptom pattern more strongly points to major depression. In addition, criteria for hypochondriasis includes a six-month period of symptoms. Further exploration of the belief that she has cancer may also suggest another modifier—major depression (single episode) with psychotic features. (**Ref. 4,** pp. 339–345, 464–465)

176. **(E)** There is some suggestion that the woman may have an obsessive–compulsive disorder but the information is insufficient. More exploration of this person's patterns of interpersonal relationships and use of defense mechanisms throughout her adult life

are necessary to determine the presence of any personality disorder. (**Ref. 4,** pp. 629–630)

177. **(E)** Delusions of cancer would make a subclassification of "with psychotic features" possible. The patient does show loss of pleasure in all activities, early morning awakening, excessive guilt, morning exacerbation, anorexia, and weight loss. Hence, she can be classified as "with melancholia." This is important pharmacologically, because these symptoms are likely to respond to antidepressants. (**Ref. 2,** p. 203)

178. **(E)** With second and subsequent attacks of major depression, it is classified as recurrent. (**Ref. 4,** p. 339)

179. **(A)** Somatic delusions pertain to the functioning of one's body. Hypochondriacal delusions are also somatic delusions when they involve specific changes in the functioning or structure of the body. Some may argue that this "belief" has reached the point of being delusional and may instead reflect a distrust of doctors or, perhaps, misunderstandings of what medicine can or cannot do. (**Ref. 4,** pp. 339–345, 462–464)

180. **(B)** Suicide risk increases with depressed mood, especially if vegetative signs are present. The topic of suicide should always be discussed with a depressed patient. (**Ref. 2,** pp. 216–217)

181. **(E)** Suicide among depressed patients is more likely at the onset or the end of a depressive episode. Thus, if the patient is becoming better or getting energized, she is in a high-risk period. Studies show that about 40% of depressed patients who commit suicide have made a previous attempt. A family history of suicide also greatly increases the risk. Although generally it is a good prognostic sign for a patient to confide suicidal ideas with her psychiatrist, this is not the case if she is not implicitly willing to disavow them. (**Ref. 2,** pp. 216–217)

182. **(E)** Married persons have the lowest suicide rates. The suicide rate for single persons is twice the rate for married persons; the suicide rate for divorced, separated, or widowed persons is 4 to 5 times higher than that of married persons. (**Ref. 1,** pp. 803–804)

183. (B) Fixation at, or regression to, the anal stage is considered important in the compulsive personality. Traits associated with the compulsive personality are emotional constriction, orderliness, parsimony, rigidity, and obstinacy. **(Ref. 1, p. 745)**

184. (C) Certainly this woman's major depression should be treated with an antidepressant; a tricyclic such as desipramine is a reasonable choice. In addition, given her somatic delusions, she should be placed on a low dose, relatively high-potency, antipsychotic, such as haloperidol. **(Ref. 1, pp. 548–551)**

185. (E) Although amitriptyline blocks the reuptake of norepinephrine, its effects are stronger in blocking the reuptake of serotonin. **(Ref. 3, p. 219)**

186. (A) Generalized anxiety disorder is characterized by excessive worry and anxiety for at least 6 months. The symptoms are persistent and present most of the time and are accompanied by at least 3 of the following symptoms: restlessness, easily fatigued, difficulty concentrating, irritability, muscle tension, or sleep disturbance. Panic disorders are discrete, not persistent, episodes. Worry in obsessive–compulsive disorder does not typically involve real life problems. In agoraphobia, the essential feature is anxiety about being in places where a person may find it difficult to escape. **(Ref. 4, pp. 396, 417–423, 432–436)**

187. (E) The symptom of anxiety may occur in a wide range of physical and mental disorders. It is important to differentiate anxiety arising from organic causes and direct the appropriate treatment toward these causes. The obsessive–compulsive personality usually does not experience significant anxiety, at least not as a presentation upon treatment, because he/she uses isolation of affect as a defense mechanism. The person with obsessive–compulsive disorder is emotionally constricted. **(Ref. 1, pp. 578–579, 745)**

188. (E) Factitious disorder with physical symptoms (Münchhausen syndrome) has been applied to people who feign a severe illness and make recurrent hospitalizations a way of life. Unlike malingerers, they do not profit economically from this. Many are exposed to dangerous diagnostic and surgical procedures. These patients frequently have close connections with people in medicine or are themselves in medically related careers. Physicians may become incensed because the feigned disease is "not real" and miss the fact that this is a very severe and disabling condition. (**Ref. 1,** p. 634; **Ref. 3,** pp. 294–295)

189. (A) The incidence of factitious disorder in men and women is unknown. Different sources, however, will suggest that one or the other has a higher incidence. (**Ref. 3,** pp. 294–295; **Ref. 4,** pp. 471–473)

190. (A) Somatization disorder is characterized by a history of many physical complaints beginning before the age of 30 and persisting for several years. Hypochondriasis is the preoccupation with the fear of having or the belief that one has a serious disease. Hypochondriasis is equally likely to afflict males and females, whereas somatization disorder is much more likely to be found in females. (**Ref. 4,** pp. 447–449, 462–465)

191. (A) Somatization disorder usually begins in the second decade and runs a fluctuating course, although the patient rarely is entirely free of symptoms. Patients lack the characteristic biological signs and symptoms of depression. Although they may include conversion phenomena in their list of complaints, the term "conversion disorder" should be reserved for those in whom conversion symptoms are the primary and predominant manifestation of illness. Hypochondriasis is characterized by the obsessive fear that one might have an illness and unrealistic interpretations of physical signs and symptoms. In factitious disorders (eg Münchhausen syndrome) and in malingering, there is a conscious and deliberate intent to produce medical signs and symptoms and to misrepresent histories. (**Ref. 1,** pp. 618, 632)

192. (C) This woman meets the criteria for panic disorder. Although she clearly is uncomfortable with and avoids driving, she does not restrict her travel or need a companion. In addition, she does not endorse a fear of being in places or situations from which escape might be difficult or embarrassing (the principal criteria for agoraphobia). (**Ref. 4,** pp. 235–239)

193. (C) The "minor" traffic accident does have a temporal relationship to the onset of symptoms. Its significance in the history as described in unclear, but of some obvious importance. None of the other items have been identified as specific problems in themselves, nor is it clear that any home issues are relevant to the problem at hand. (**Ref. 4,** pp. 29–30, 397)

194. (E) Although less likely, further information to rule these out is needed. Appropriate questions for each would be: Social phobia—is there something about the social situations that makes this woman feel "on stage"? Somatization disorder—are there any more GI symptoms or pain? Posttraumatic stress disorder—the patient has many associated symptoms to this disorder, but are there any recurrences (nightmares, flashbacks) of the accident? Any numbing of affect? And finally, substance-induced anxiety disorder—is there any history of caffeine, alcohol, amphetamines, or diet pill use or abuse? (**Ref. 4,** pp. 400–401)

195. (C) She has moderate symptomatology but has managed to cope well. Although her external social functioning would be more indicative of a GAF of about 80, her internal distress is the predominant consideration in this case. (**Ref. 4,** pp. 30–32)

196. (D) Trichotillomania is an irresistible urge to pull out one's own hair, resulting in noticeable hair loss. There is tension preceding the behavior and relief associated with the commission of the act. (**Ref. 1,** pp. 724–725; **Ref. 4,** pp. 618–621)

197. (A) Axis II refers to developmental and personality disorders. This patient presents substantial evidence (via his MMPI) of an obsessive–compulsive personality disorder. (**Ref. 1,** p. 745)

198. (B) These disorders are characterized by the failure to resist an impulse or drive to act in a specific way that is harmful to oneself or others. (**Ref. 4,** p. 609)

199. (E) None of the above has been consistently shown to be the best treatment for this condition. All have been tried with variable results. (**Ref. 1,** p. 725)

200. (B)   201. (A)   202. (B)   203. (B)   Seen in cluster B are behaviors that are dramatic, emotional, and erratic. The use of acting out as a defense mechanism is seen in the cluster B personality disorders (histrionic, narcissistic, antisocial, and borderline). Odd but not clearly delusional thinking is seen in cluster A. The belief in "the little signal" suggests some oddities in thinking. (**Refs. 1,** pp. 731, 736–742; **Ref. 3,** pp. 172–174)

5

Medical Psychiatric Illness
Kathryn C. Krieg

DIRECTIONS (Questions 1 through 28): Each of the questions or incomplete statements below is followed by five suggested answers or completions. Select the ONE that is best in each case.

---

1. The DSM–IV diagnosis "psychological factor affecting medical condition" is characterized by which of the following?
    A. a general medical condition is judged to be causing a mental disorder through a direct physiological mechanism
    B. a substance use disorder is adversely affecting or causing a general medical condition
    C. psychological or behavioral factors adversely affect a general medical condition by influencing the development of the condition, by interfering with the treatment of the condition, by constituting additional health risks, or by precipitating or exacerbating the symptoms of the medical condition
    D. it is synonymous with somatoform disorders
    E. noncompliance with medical treatment is the major focus of clinic attention

2. The most effective treatment of the mildly to moderately obese individual is
   A. gastroplasty surgery
   B. very low-calorie diet
   C. inpatient hospital treatment program
   D. residential treatment program
   E. self-help or commercial program with continuous care

3. Psychotherapeutic interventions in patients with ulcerative colitis
   A. are most effective when combined with behavioral approaches such as biofeedback and relaxation techniques
   B. are most effective when patients are confronted about their maladaptive behaviors
   C. can significantly improve the rate of mortality from illness
   D. can decrease symptomatology and improve overall bowel function and adaptation to illness
   E. are generally felt to be ineffective

4. Which of the following statements is true regarding anorexia nervosa?
   A. the following subtypes have been identified: restricting type and binge-eating/purging type
   B. the following types have been identified: purging type and nonpurging type
   C. diagnostic criteria include severe anorexia or appetite loss
   D. diagnostic criteria include a weight loss leading to maintenance of body weight less than 75% expected for age and height
   E. extensive weight loss often leads to fatigue and hypersomnia

5. A 70-year-old married man, father of two, has been hospitalized for a course of treatment for prostatic cancer. Test results reveal metastatic disease to the bone, brain, and liver. Which of the following is the MOST appropriate behavior for the patient's physician in conveying the bad news? The physician should
   A. discuss the test results individually with the patient on morning rounds
   B. make arrangements to sit down with the patient, his spouse, and other family members to discuss the findings and treatment

C. set aside time for a lengthy detailed discussion initially, in order to avoid the need for ongoing discussions

D. discuss the findings with the patient's spouse and other family members alone, since recent studies show that most patients prefer not to be informed of a diagnosis of advanced malignancy

E. request that a psychiatric consultant convey the bad news to the patient

6. Recent studies of stress-related immunologic changes have revealed that

A. stressful stimuli do not affect susceptibility to bacterial and viral infections

B. immunologic changes have been found in patients with mood disorders, personality disorders, and schizophrenia, when compared to normal controls

C. minor stressors such as marital discord, unemployment, or financial difficulties do not appear to have an effect on the immune response

D. during bereavement, surviving spouses show a significantly decreased T cell proliferation

E. psychoactive medications do not appear to alter immune function to any significant degree

7. Cardiologists Meyer Friedman and Ray Rosenman have described a specific behavior pattern called type A. Which of the following statements is true regarding type A behavior?

A. individuals with type A behavior are more successful than those with type B behavior

B. the most important aspects of type A behavior in regard to risk of coronary artery disease are time urgency and competitive hostility

C. the degree of type A behavior correlates directly with the degree of coronary artery narrowing seen on angiography

D. individuals with type A behavior are also at higher risk of developing rheumatoid arthritis than those with type B behavior

E. type A behavior also favors the development of cardiac arrhythmias

8. According to a well-known study by Thomas H. Holmes and Richard Rahe, onset of medical or psychiatric illness is preceded by which of the following in regard to life events and life crises?
   A. a marked decrease in number
   B. an increase in number
   C. little or no change in number or quality
   D. considerable variation in number
   E. a change in the quality

9. Which of the following factors is most strongly correlated with good compliance (adherence to physician recommendations)?
   A. type A personality
   B. increased complexity of medication regimen
   C. female sex
   D. higher socioeconomic status
   E. subjective feeling of distress or illness

10. When a terminal illness occurs in an individual, which of the following is often observed in the family members?
   A. remission of any preexisting psychopathology
   B. intensification of family conflicts
   C. solidification of roles
   D. transient psychotic episodes
   E. stable patterns of maintaining discipline

11. The MOST important clinical application of biofeedback is in the treatment of
   A. headache symptoms
   B. peptic ulcer disease
   C. transient psychotic episodes
   D. asthma
   E. Graves' disease

12. Which of the following statements is TRUE regarding the placebo response?
   A. approximately 5% of persons in pain will obtain relief from an inert substance as if they were given an analgesic
   B. the placebo response is a normal aspect of personality and cannot be linked with any type of psychopathology
   C. following surgery, about 10% of patients obtain pain relief from injections of saline

    D. the placebo trial is a useful method of separating psychogenic from organic pain

    E. the placebo response is seen commonly in individuals with antisocial personality disorder

13. Patients with rheumatoid arthritis
    A. are usually refractory to psychotherapeutic interventions
    B. often demonstrate a type A pattern of behavior
    C. have often experienced psychological trauma prior to the onset of symptoms
    D. are often alexithymic
    E. are often self-sacrificing, masochistic, inhibited, and perfectionistic

14. A 32-year-old man complains of headache pain in the area of his left eye, extending to the left side of his face. The pain began the day following his friend's bachelor party; it caused him to be awakened from his nap and has been present daily for the last two weeks. The MOST likely diagnosis is
    A. migraine headache
    B. hangover
    C. tension headache
    D. cluster headache
    E. postconcussion syndrome

15. A 45-year-old woman received an aortic valve replacement two days prior to psychiatric consultation. The procedure lasted about one hour longer than expected but was otherwise unremarkable. The CCU staff initially noted that she was anxious, depressed, and irritable. She now complains that the walls are closing in on her and claims that she is being held against her will as part of a communist plot. The MOST appropriate diagnosis is
    A. major depressive disorder, severe, with psychotic features
    B. schizophrenia
    C. postoperative psychosis
    D. brief reactive psychosis
    E. postcardiotomy delirium

16. The patient described in the preceding question is becoming agitated and has pulled out a pacemaker wire and an endotracheal tube. While other work-up is proceeding, which medication regimen would be MOST useful in sedating this patient?
    A. chlorpromazine, 100 mg IV
    B. haloperidol, 10 mg IM
    C. pancuronium bromide, 3 mg IV
    D. haloperidol, 10 mg IV
    E. morphine sulfate, 4 mg IV

17. Which of the following etiologic factors is MOST likely to be involved in the pathogenesis of the condition of the patient in Question 15?
    A. CCU environment
    B. preoperative organic brain disease
    C. history of schizophrenia
    D. high level of preoperative anxiety
    E. sleep deprivation

18. Which of the following medications is correctly paired with the psychiatric symptom it is likely to cause?
    A. oral contraceptives/psychosis
    B. reserpine/mania
    C. sympathomimetics/depression
    D. theophylline/mania
    E. methyldopa/depression

19. In the development of peptic ulcer disease, Weiner and co-workers postulated an interaction between specific psychological patterns of dependency conflict and
    A. level of pepsinogen secretion
    B. salicylate levels
    C. number of pack years of cigarette smoking
    D. daily caffeine consumption
    E. ulcerogenic diet

20. When treating a terminally ill patient, it is important to remember that the Kubler–Ross stages
  A. are a simple construct that adequately explains the coping behavior of the dying
  B. are universal coping responses unaffected by previous experiences or cultural beliefs
  C. represent normal reactions to loss and may occur simultaneously, disappear and reappear, or occur in any order
  D. follow a linear progression, with the patient preceding from one stage directly to the next
  E. do not include fear and anxiety because these emotions occur infrequently in terminally ill patients

21. Psychological accommodation to impending death
  A. is not possible in children under the age of 13
  B. maximizes the patient's dignity
  C. promotes long-term psychological scarring in family members
  D. contradicts the wishes of most patients
  E. should generally be avoided

22. Which of the following statements is TRUE regarding coping and adaptation to chronic medical illness?
  A. brief psychotic episodes are common
  B. MMPI profiles reveal elevated scores in depression, hysteria, and sociopathy
  C. suicidal behavior is seen frequently in hospitalized medical and surgical patients
  D. psychiatric disorders occur in about 5% of medical inpatients
  E. it is useful to understand how a patient experienced previous illnesses

23. Which of the following pairs of medical disorders and psychiatric presentations is correctly matched?
  A. hypothyroidism/panic attacks
  B. hyperthyroidism/dementia
  C. hyponatremia/mania
  D. vitamin B_{12} deficiency/dementia
  E. hypoglycemia/psychosis

24. Which of these factors may reduce a patient's compliance with medical regimens?
   A. physician enthusiasm
   B. recommendations from several clinicians about medications
   C. short physician waiting room time
   D. informing family and support persons about the medication
   E. providing the patient with written instructions

25. In studying human reactions to overwhelming trauma, which of the following is the BEST predictor of the development of post-traumatic stress disorder?
   A. youthful age
   B. poor physical health
   C. recent excessive alcohol intake
   D. type A behavior
   E. unemployment

26. Which of the following antidepressant medications appears to possess a "therapeutic window"?
   A. fluoxetine
   B. doxepin
   C. imipramine
   D. nortriptyline
   E. buproprion

27. Which of the following is an example of a cause of reversible dementia?
   A. primary degenerative dementia of the Alzheimer type
   B. pellagra
   C. schizophrenia
   D. multi-infarct dementia
   E. Pick's disease

28. Which of the following sets of laboratory results would be MOST consistent with a diagnosis of alcoholism?
   A. elevated bilirubin; microcytic anemia
   B. elevated serum glutamic oxatoacetic transaminase (SGOT); vitamin B_{12} deficiency
   C. elevated gamma-glutamyl transpeptidase (GGT); macrocytosis

D. elevated serum glutamic pyruvic transaminase (SGPT); folate toxicity

E. blood alcohol level; iron deficiency

DIRECTIONS (Questions 29 and 30): This section consists of a clinical situation followed by a series of questions. Study the situation and select the ONE best answer to each question following it.

A 76-year-old widow presents to her family physician stating that her skin has been infested by spiders. She points to numerous excoriations on all four extremities and states that these are the areas of infestation. She describes in great detail cleaning an oven, which was filled with spider eggs, and notes that her symptoms began after this event. She has tried numerous over-the-counter and home remedies without success. She now wonders if she might need to see a "skin doctor."

The patient is polite and cooperative during the examination. There is no evidence of hallucinations or disorganized thoughts. Mental status examination, neurologic studies, and laboratory screening failed to reveal evidence of any organic disorder.

29. Her MOST likely diagnosis is
    A. delusional disorder, somatic type
    B. schizophreniform disorder
    C. alcohol-induced psychotic disorder with delusions
    D. Münchhausen's syndrome
    E. conversion disorder

30. The MOST effective treatment for this patient would be
    A. psychoanalysis
    B. dermatology consultation
    C. confrontation about her attention-seeking behavior
    D. biofeedback
    E. pimozide

DIRECTIONS (Questions 31 through 42): Each group of questions below consists of lettered headings followed by a list of numbered words, phrases, or statements. For each numbered word, phrase, or statement, select the ONE lettered heading that is most closely associated with it. Each lettered heading may be selected once, more than once, or not at all.

Questions 31 through 37

    A. agranulocytosis
    B. hypothyroidism
    C. tyramine-induced hypertensive crisis
    D. anorgasmia
    E. priapism

31. Phenelzine

32. Clozapine

33. Paroxetine

34. Carbamazepine

35. Sertraline

36. Trazodone

37. Lithium carbonate

Questions 38 through 42

    A. generalized seizures–absences (petit mal)
    B. partial seizures–simple
    C. partial seizures–complex
    D. pseudoseizure

38. Patient has conscious control over symptoms

39. Onset usually during childhood

40. Most common form of epilepsy in adults

41. Ten percent to thirty percent of patients also have psychotic symptoms

42. Ethosuximide is the treatment drug of choice

Medical Psychiatric Illness

Explanatory Answers

1. **(C)** Answer A describes the diagnostic category of mental disorder due to general medical condition. Answer B describes a situation in which mental disorder due to general medical condition AND substance use disorder would be coded on axis I. Somoatoform disorders (answer D) do not involve a general medical condition that can account for the physical symptoms. When noncompliance with medical treatment is the major focus of clinical attention (answer E), the diagnostic category noncompliance with treatment is used. (**Ref. 4,** pp. 675–678)

2. **(E)** Measures listed in answers A, B, C, D are best reserved for severely overweight patients or those who have failed other treatment strategies. Mildly to moderately overweight obese individuals do best with programs which gradually modify maladaptive eating and exercise behaviors. Recent research also indicates that weight loss is better maintained with long-term continuous care. (**Ref. 3,** pp. 681–686)

3. **(D)** Nonconfrontive, supportive psychotherapy is indicated during acute ulcerative colitis, with interpretative psychotherapy during the quiescent periods. Such an approach has been effective in decreasing symptomatology and in improving well-being. (**Ref. 1,** pp. 760–761)

4. (A) The DSM–IV diagnostic category of anorexia nervosa has been divided into subtypes of restricting type and binge-eating/purging type. The purging type and nonpurging type distinctions are for bulimia nervosa. The term anorexia is a misnomer, since true loss of appetite is rare. Diagnostic criteria include a weight loss leading to maintenance of body weight less than 85% expected for age and height. Patients with anorexia nervosa often appear to have excessive energy and often suffer from insomnia. (**Ref. 4,** pp. 539–545)

5. (B) Studies have shown that patients and families informed of bad news simultaneously have fewer emotional difficulties. Communicating a diagnosis is best done briefly, leaving the opportunity for ongoing dialogue with the patient and family. Most studies asking whether or not patients wish to be told the truth about malignancy show an overwhelming desire for truth. (**Ref. 3,** pp. 599–601)

6. (D) Immunologic changes in response to life stress have been observed in both human and animal studies. Patients with major depressive disorder have decreased T cell proliferation and an overall decrease in lymphocytes. Abnormal immune function has also been seen in some schizophrenic patients. Many commonly prescribed psychoactive drugs alter various parameters of immune cell function. (**Ref. 1,** p. 146)

7. (B) According to cardiologist Meyer Friedman, the most important aspects of the type A behavior pattern are time urgency and competitive hostility. Although type A individuals have an ardent desire to achieve, they are actually less successful than type B individuals. Type A behavior is a major risk factor (along with cholesterol, hypertension, smoking, and family history) for the development of coronary artery disease. It is not predictive of the degree of coronary narrowing, development of cardiac arrhythmias, or any other medical condition. (**Ref. 1,** pp. 226, 758)

8. (B) Using the Holmes and Rahe Schedule of Recent Events, it has been shown that illness onset is preceded by an accumulation of life events. (**Ref. 1,** p. 200)

9. **(E)** An increased complexity of the regimen appears to be associated with noncompliance. There is no clear association between compliance and the patient's sex, marital status, race, religion, or socioeconomic status. A highly significant factor in compliance seems to be the patient's subjective feeling of distress or illness. **(Ref. 1,** pp. 11–12)

10. **(B)** At times of great external stress, such as the impending death of a family member, family conflicts may intensify. Reevaluation and changes in family member roles, as well as changes in patterns of maintaining discipline, are commonly seen. **(Ref. 1,** pp. 77–78)

11. **(A)** The most important and common clinical application of biofeedback has been in the treatment of headache symptoms. Short-term efficacy has also been documented for hypertension, some cardiac arrhythmias, and Raynaud's phenomenon. **(Ref. 3,** pp. 496–497)

12. **(B)** Approximately 30% to 40% of any population in pain will obtain relief from an inert substance. The placebo trial is of no value in separating psychogenic from organic pain. **(Ref. 1,** p. 1013; **Ref. 3,** pp. 656–660)

13. **(C)** Studies have failed to show any characteristic premorbid personality type in patients with rheumatoid arthritis. Psychological stress may predispose patients to rheumatoid arthritis. Psychotherapy is a useful adjunct to medical treatment. **(Ref. 1,** p. 761)

14. **(D)** Cluster headache generally begins between the ages of 20 and 40. Men are affected more commonly than women. Pain typically is in the area of the orbit, but may affect adjacent areas. Cluster headaches typically awaken the patient during REM sleep; alcohol is a common precipitant. **(Ref. 1,** p. 714)

15. **(E)** Postcardiotomy delirium is the most common psychiatric phenomena associated with cardiac surgery. Impaired orientation, memory, perception, and attention are noted. Since reality testing also is impaired, delusions and hallucinations may occur. **(Ref. 3,** pp. 131–132)

16. **(D)** Chlorpromazine can abruptly decrease total peripheral resistance and cardiac output due to potent alpha-adrenergic receptor antagonism. Haloperidol may be poorly absorbed IM, and IM injections may add to the patient's paranoid thoughts. Pancuronium bromide may prolong the use of mechanical ventilation and increase the risk of respiratory compromise. Morphine sulfate will be useful only if pain is the cause of the agitation. **(Ref. 3,** pp. 132–133)

17. **(B)** History of schizophrenia alone does not predispose a patient to delirium following surgery. Preoperative anxiety has some correlation with delirium but is less important than organic factors. CCU environment and sleep deprivation have been held responsible for delirium in the past, but they are not as significant as organic factors. **(Ref. 2,** pp. 1196–1197)

18. **(E)** Methyldopa and reserpine are antihypertensive medications that may cause depression. Oral contraceptive medications may also cause depression. Sympathomimetics are most likely to cause anxiety or mania. Theophylline is most likely to cause anxiety. **(Ref. 3,** p. 602)

19. **(A)** Weiner and Mirsky measured pepsinogen levels and administered a number of psychological tests to healthy men. In combination, high pepsinogen levels plus specific psychological patterns could predict the development of ulcer disease. **(Ref. 1,** pp. 753–760)

20. **(C)** This stage construct is too simplistic to explain all of the complexities of coping behavior in the dying. Coping behavior is also shaped by previous experiences with death and cultural beliefs. It is most useful to regard the stages as normal reactions to loss, which may overlap, disappear and reappear, or occur in any order. **(Ref. 3,** p. 599)

21. **(B)** At about age 9 or 10, most children are able to conceptualize death as something that can happen to a child as well as to a parent. Most patients and their family members wish their physicians to be truthful with them regarding the facts of a terminal condition. **(Ref. 1,** pp. 77–80)

22. (E) Studies show that up to 65% of medical inpatients have psychiatric disorders, most commonly anxiety, depression, disorientation. Illness behavior and the sick role are affected by a person's previous experience with illness and cultural beliefs about disease. **(Ref. 1,** pp. 1, 771–775)

23. (D) The most common psychiatric presentation for hypothyroidism is a retarded depression. Hyperthyroidism most commonly presents with anxiety, panic attacks, or agitated depression. Hyponatremia can cause either depression or psychosis. Hypoglycemia can cause anxiety or panic attacks. Vitamin B_{12} deficiency can present with either psychotic symptoms or dementia. **(Ref. 3,** pp. 604–605)

24. (B) Involving multiple clinicians in medication recommendations may reduce compliance. All other factors listed can enhance compliance. **(Ref. 1,** pp. 11–12)

25. (C) The predisposing vulnerability factors that appear to play primary roles in the development of posttraumatic stress disorder include such items as presence of childhood trauma; borderline, paranoid, dependent, or antisocial personality disorder traits; inadequate support system; recent stressful life changes; and recent excessive alcohol intake. **(Ref 1,** p. 607)

26. (D) Methods are available to evaluate blood levels for most tricyclic antidepressants. These generally have not been used, with the exception of nortriptyline. Nortriptyline appears to possess a "therapeutic window," meaning that depressed patients do best when they have nortriptyline blood levels of 50 to 150 mg/mL. **(Ref. 1,** p. 285)

27. (B) Vitamin deficiency states, such as vitamin B_{12} deficiency, thiamine deficiency, and niacin deficiency (or pellagra) are examples of causes of reversible dementia. At this time, Alzheimer's disease, Pick's disease, and multi-infarct dementia are irreversible. Schizophrenia is in the differential diagnosis of dementia. **(Ref. 1,** pp. 345–349)

28. (C) Useful laboratory findings in confirming the diagnosis of alcoholism include blood alcohol level; elevated liver enzymes, particularly GGT; macrocytosis; and folate deficiency. Radiology studies often reveal fractures, subdural hematomas, pneumonia, and other pulmonary problems. (**Ref. 1,** p. 401)

29. **(A)**   The patient described best meets criteria for a diagnosis of delusional disorder, somatic type. She demonstrates nonbizarre delusions, with normal behavior apart from the delusions. She does not meet the criteria for schizophrenia or a mood disorder and has no evidence of a medical condition. (**Ref. 1,** pp. 503–509)

30. **(E)**   Some investigators have indicated that pimozide may be particularly effective in delusional disorder, especially in patients with somatic delusions. (**Ref. 1,** pp. 510–512)

31. **(C),   32. (A),   33. (D),   34. (A),   35. (D),   36. (E), 37. (B),**   When patients taking monoamine oxidase inhibitors ingest foods rich in tyramine, they are at risk for a life-threatening hypertensive reaction. Agranulocytosis occurs in 1% to 2% of all patients taking clozapine. Severe blood dyscrasias (including agranulocytosis) occur in about 1 in 20,000 patients treated with carbamezepine. Serotonin-specific reuptake inhibitors cause sexual side effects such as anorgasmia, impotence, and delayed ejaculation in about 5% of patients treated. Trazodone is associated with a rare occurrence of priapism or prolonged erection. Lithium causes a benign, transient diminution in the concentration or circulating thyroid hormones. (**Ref. 1,** pp. 888–1015)

38. **(D),   39. (A),   40. (C),   41. (C),   42. (A)**   A   pseudoseizure is that in which a patient has conscious control over mimicking the symptoms of a seizure. Absences (petit mal) seizures usually begin during childhood, and treatment drugs of choice include ethosuximide, valproric acid, and trimethadione. Complex partial epilepsy is the most common form of epilepsy in adults, and between 10% and 30% of patients also have psychotic symptoms. (**Ref. 1,** pp. 364–368)

6

Treatment

Gunnar Larson
Robert Chayer

DIRECTIONS (Questions 1 through 61): Each of the questions or incomplete statements below is followed by five suggested answers or completions. Select the ONE that is best in each case.

1. The mechanism of action of typical antipsychotic agents is thought to result primarily from
   A. blockade of dopamine D-1 receptors
   B. blockade of dopamine D-2 receptors
   C. blockade of serotonin 5-HT1 reuptake
   D. blockade of serotonin 5-HT2 reuptake
   E. blockade of acetylcholine release

2. Tacrine is characterized by all of the following EXCEPT
   A. reversible inhibition of acetylcholine-sterase
   B. lowers acetylcholine concentrations in the synaptic cleft
   C. increases hepatic enzymes
   D. used in treatment of mildly to moderately ill patients with Alzheimer's dementia
   E. can cause nausea, vomiting, diarrhea

3. Anticholinergic toxicity is characterized by all of the following EXCEPT
  A. agitation
  B. disorientation
  C. urinary hesitancy
  D. impairment of immediate memory
  E. olfactory hallucinations

4. All of the following are true of tardive dyskinesia EXCEPT
  A. it frequently first becomes evident during dosage reduction or withdrawal of antipsychotic therapy
  B. it is a movement disorder
  C. it occurs only with antipsychotic medications
  D. it can be treatment resistant
  E. it usually does not occur within the first few months of antipsychotic exposure

5. An adequate trial of an antidepressant is now considered to be
  A. at least one to two weeks after starting medication
  B. at least one to two weeks after reaching the suggested therapeutic dose
  C. at least two to four weeks after reaching the suggested therapeutic dose
  D. at least four to six weeks after reaching the suggested therapeutic dose
  E. at least eight to twelve weeks after reaching the suggested therapeutic dose

6. Symptoms of benzodiazepine withdrawal include all of the following EXCEPT
  A. diaphoresis
  B. restlessness
  C. hallucinations
  D. hyperacusis
  E. delusions

7. All of the following are considered accurate clinical guidelines in using antidepressants EXCEPT
    A. an adequate trial should last at least four to six weeks after reaching the suggested therapeutic dose
    B. when the acute episode is in remission, the patient should be maintained on a more tolerable lower dose for at least six to twelve months
    C. the more episodes of depression a patient has, the more likely a recurrence is
    D. for patients experiencing their first episode, a family history is the best predictor of future episodes
    E. after three or more episodes of depression coming at more frequent intervals, indefinite long-term therapy with an anti-depressant should be considered

8. All of the following statements are true with regard to fluoxetine and sertraline EXCEPT
    A. fluoxetine may take several weeks to reach its steady state concentration
    B. sertraline inhibits the hepatic P-450 oxidase system and can result in a four- to six-fold increase in other drugs, including tricyclic antidepressants
    C. patients cannot be switched from fluoxetine to an MAOI until at least five weeks have passed since stopping fluoxetine
    D. sertraline has no significant active metabolites
    E. sertraline is a four to five times more potent inhibitor of serotonin reuptake than fluoxetine

9. Early evidence of lithium toxicity includes all of the following EXCEPT
    A. ataxia
    B. nausea
    C. coarse tremors
    D. seizures
    E. listlessness

10. In the treatment of acute mania, the blood level of lithium should be
    A. 0.1 to 0.2 mEq/L
    B. 0.2 to 0.5 mEq/L
    C. 0.8 to 1.2 mEq/L

D. 1.2 to 2.4 mEq/L
E. 2.4 to 3.0 mEq/L

11. Neuroleptic malignant syndrome (NMS) is characterized by all of the following EXCEPT
    A. hyperthermia and autonomic instability
    B. muscle rigidity
    C. a mortality rate of approximately 20% if untreated
    D. results from a hyperdopaminergic state
    E. altered consciousness/delirium

12. Valproic acid is characterized by all of the following statements with regard to its clinical usage EXCEPT
    A. it is an effective anticonvulsant
    B. it is an effective antimanic agent
    C. it is an effective alternative antipsychotic agent
    D. it may play a useful role in patients with regard to benzodiazepine discontinuation after dependence has developed
    E. it may play a role in treating panic attacks

13. All of the following are potential side effects of lithium EXCEPT
    A. decreased urine output
    B. rashes
    C. ECG changes
    D. granulocytosis
    E. hypoparathyroidism

14. All of the following can commonly occur as a side effect of lithium EXCEPT
    A. T wave flattening
    B. T wave inversion
    C. premature ventricular contractions
    D. first degree AV block
    E. U waves

15. A violent reaction to naloxone (Narcan) characterized by lacrimation, yawning, pupillary dilatation, restlessness, and sweating suggests
   A. a heroin dependence
   B. a cannabis dependence
   C. an amphetamine dependence
   D. an alcohol dependence
   E. hypoglycemia

16. The only absolute contraindication to electroconvulsive therapy (ECT) is
   A. a threatened retinal detachment
   B. glaucoma
   C. an aortic aneurysm
   D. a brain mass with increased intracranial pressure
   E. myocardial disease

17. Which of the following antipsychotics CANNOT cross the placenta?
   A. haloperidol
   B. chlorpromazine
   C. fluphenazine
   D. perphenazine
   E. none of the above

18. All of the following types of data are used in biofeedback EXCEPT
   A. electromyography (EMG)
   B. peripheral skin temperature
   C. electroencephalography (EEG)
   D. dexamethasone suppression test (DST)
   E. galvanic skin response

19. All of the following statements are true regarding benzodiazepines EXCEPT
   A. benzodiazepines bind to a site on GABA-a receptors distinct from the GABA recognition site
   B. benzodiazepines decrease the affinity of the GABA-a receptor for GABA
   C. alcohol also affects GABA-a receptor function

D. cimetidine may increase benzodiazepine blood levels
E. benzodiazepines interact with few other drugs with the exception of other CNS depressants

20. As opposed to respondent or Pavlovian conditioning, in operant conditioning
    A. responses are conditioned by consequent response
    B. responses are conditioned by antecedent stimuli
    C. behavior is strengthened by absence of response
    D. behavior is strengthened by pairing of a neutral stimulus
    E. none of the above

21. All of the following are examples of countertransference EXCEPT
    A. forgetting a patient's appointment
    B. arguing with a patient
    C. dreaming of a patient
    D. desiring to ask favors of a patient
    E. the patient's forgetting an appointment

22. All of the following are true of tricyclic coma EXCEPT
    A. there is no need for hospitalization
    B. it is of short duration—24 hours or less
    C. death typically is due to cardiac arrhythmia
    D. respiratory depression is common
    E. recovery is possible

23. Crisis stabilization techniques include all of the following EXCEPT
    A. emphasis on current problems and functioning
    B. mobilization of social support systems
    C. rapid symptom relief
    D. personality change
    E. decision counseling

24. Clozapine is an atypical antipsychotic characterized by the following EXCEPT
   A. it is an effective antipsychotic for 50% to 70% of nonresponders to standard antipsychotics
   B. starting dose should be 25 mg/day to minimize orthostatic hypotension
   C. approximately 1% of patients on clozapine may develop agranulocytosis
   D. the risk of developing tardive dyskinesia appears reduced or nonexistent compared to standard antipsychotics
   E. there is a dose-related increased risk of seizures

25. The use of anti-parkinsonian agents is indicated for the treatment of which of the following side effects of haloperidol?
   A. dystonia
   B. sedation
   C. confusion
   D. postural hypotension
   E. none of the above

26. All of the following statements are true with regard to suicide risk for psychiatric patients EXCEPT
   A. middle-aged patients have a higher suicide risk
   B. suicide is preceded by an undesirable life event
   C. suicide occurs more often in women
   D. psychiatric patients have a higher incidence of self injury
   E. whites are at higher risk

27. All of the following endocrine side effects have been reported in patients on antipsychotics EXCEPT
   A. false-positive pregnancy tests
   B. diabetes
   C. delayed ejaculation
   D. increased lactation
   E. gynecomastia

28. A 22-year-old female is brought to the emergency room after ingesting several handfuls of an unknown prescription medication. On arrival, she is delirious and agitated. Physical examination reveals dilated pupils; warm, dry skin; depressed bowel sounds; tachycardia, and hyperreflexia. The ingested medication MOST likely was

A. haloperidol
B. fluoxetine
C. diazepam
D. lithium
E. imipramine

29. All of the following statements are true with regard to the efficacy of antipsychotics in treating acute psychosis EXCEPT

A. no standard antipsychotic has been demonstrated to be more effective than another
B. benzodiazepines can prove a useful adjunct to antipsychotics in treating acute agitation
C. there was no significant placebo response in an NIMH collaborative study when looking at psychotic patients who were much improved or in remission
D. parenteral antipsychotics are absorbed more quickly than oral preparations
E. given in equal milligram doses, parenteral preparations result in higher blood levels

30. Propranolol has all of the following psychiatric indications EXCEPT

A. akathisia
B. violence associated with antisocial personality disorder
C. TCA-induced fine, rapid tremor
D. rage attacks and aggression in autistic disorder
E. lithium-induced tremor

31. Standard or typical antipsychotics have among their side effects all of the following EXCEPT

A. exanthematous biliary cirrhosis
B. retinitis pigmentosa
C. blue-grey metallic caste to the skin in areas exposed to the sun
D. agranulocytosis
E. increased seizure threshold

32. Panic disorder can be effectively managed with all of the following EXCEPT
- **A.** imipramine
- **B.** monoamine oxidase inhibitors
- **C.** lithium carbonate
- **D.** alprazolam
- **E.** cognitive behavioral therapy

33. A 37-year-old female is referred to a psychiatrist because she is convinced that her liver is diseased. Despite several unremarkable GI workups and repeated assurances, she is preoccupied with her "cancer" and has completely stopped eating. The pharmacologic treatment of choice is
- **A.** pimozide
- **B.** lorazepam
- **C.** desipramine
- **D.** carbamazepine
- **E.** phenelzine

34. Therapeutic uses of lithium include all of the following EXCEPT
- **A.** maintenance therapy for bipolar disorder
- **B.** potentiation of tricyclic antidepressants
- **C.** treatment of cyclothymia
- **D.** treatment of schizoaffective disorder
- **E.** treatment of schizophrenia

35. Psychiatric uses of beta-blocking agents (beta-adrenergic receptor antagonists) include the management of all of the following EXCEPT
- **A.** performance anxiety
- **B.** tardive dyskinesia
- **C.** neuroleptic-induced akathisia
- **D.** lithium tremor
- **E.** impulsive violence with organic brain syndromes

36. All of the following are effective in the treatment of obsessive–compulsive disorder EXCEPT
- **A.** clomipramine
- **B.** exposure techniques

C. methylphenidate
D. fluoxetine
E. response prevention techniques

37. All of the following are indications for the use of psychostimulants EXCEPT
    A. treatment of morbid obesity
    B. treatment of attention-deficit hyperactivity disorder in children
    C. treatment of apathy and withdrawal in the medically ill and elderly
    D. potentiation of narcotic analgesics
    E. narcolepsy

38. Which of the following statements is TRUE regarding the use of behavior therapy in the treatment of obesity?
    A. The majority of people maintain clinically significant weight loss for more than one year after treatment
    B. Distracting activities while eating (eg, reading, watching TV) tend to reduce caloric intake
    C. Adjunctive exercise programs result in increased caloric intake and subsequent weight gain
    D. Self-monitoring behaviors (eg, food diaries) are beneficial for weight management
    E. Behavior treatments are more effective in adult-onset versus child-onset obesity

39. A 46-year-old male with a longstanding history of daily alcohol use presents with delirium, ophthalmoplegia, and ataxia. The immediate treatment of choice is
    A. chlordiazepoxide, 100 mg IM
    B. thiamine, 100 mg IM
    C. benztropine, 1 mg IM
    D. D5W, 250 cc IV bolus
    E. close monitoring of vital signs

40. Hypnosis has been found effective in the treatment of all of the following EXCEPT
   A. dissociative disorders
   B. phobias
   C. conversion reactions
   D. pain management
   E. schizophrenia

41. Which of the following statements is TRUE regarding buspirone?
   A. it exhibits cross-tolerance with benzodiazepines
   B. it is not effective in suppression of alcohol withdrawal symptoms
   C. it exhibits cross-tolerance with barbiturates
   D. anxiolytic effects occur within one to two days
   E. physiologic dependency can develop

42. Electroconvulsive therapy (ECT) presently is the MOST effective treatment available for
   A. tardive dyskinesia
   B. major depressive episode with melancholia or psychotic features
   C. obsessive–compulsive disorder
   D. agoraphobia
   E. schizophrenia

43. Pharmacologic agents found clinically beneficial in the treatment of bulimia nervosa include
   A. antidepressants
   B. anticonvulsants
   C. antipsychotics
   D. barbiturates
   E. none of the above

44. Management of the violent patient may include all of the following EXCEPT
   A. removal of weapons
   B. seclusion in a safe setting
   C. use of beta-blocking agents
   D. medical investigation to rule out underlying organic disease
   E. constant reassurance

45. All of the following are normal changes affecting pharmacokinetics in the elderly patient EXCEPT
   A. the amount of GI absorption is significantly decreased
   B. albumin levels are decreased
   C. first-pass hepatic extraction is decreased
   D. total body water is reduced
   E. glomerular filtration rate (GFR) is decreased

46. The symptom LEAST likely to respond to an antidepressant medication is
   A. appetite disturbance
   B. sleep disturbance
   C. decreased energy
   D. diurnal mood variation
   E. low self-esteem

47. Treatment-resistant patients with all of the following conditions are likely to respond to psychosurgery EXCEPT
   A. major depression with vegetative signs
   B. obsessive–compulsive disorder
   C. severe chronic pain
   D. debilitating anxiety
   E. bipolar disorder

48. Systematic desensitization includes all of the following EXCEPT
   A. progressive relaxation techniques
   B. construction of a hierarchy of feared situations
   C. visual imagery
   D. gradual mastery of anxiety-provoking situations
   E. implosion

49. Cognitive therapy
   A. is especially effective with manic patients
   B. typically involves long-term treatment
   C. is best administered in an inpatient setting
   D. is based on the premise that thoughts influence mood
   E. includes aversive conditioning techniques

50. In the structural family therapy approach, the therapist
  A. assumes a passive and nondirective role
  B. focuses on boundary issues between parents and children
  C. interprets unconscious thoughts and behaviors
  D. explains current behaviors in the context of past development
  E. separates children from parents during therapy sessions

51. In individuals predisposed to panic, all of the following will likely precipitate a panic attack EXCEPT
  A. barbiturates
  B. yohimbine
  C. carbon dioxide
  D. lactate
  E. caffeine

52. The therapeutic plasma level of carbamazepine for the treatment of partial complex seizures is
  A. 0.5 to 3.0 mg/L
  B. 3.0 to 6.0 mg/L
  C. 6.0 to 12.0 mg/L
  D. 12.0 to 15.0 mg/L
  E. none of the above

53. When a patient is angry about treatment, which of the following interventions is LEAST helpful?
  A. listening to the patient
  B. discussing areas in which the patient's expectations and the physician's treatment do not match
  C. being empathetic to the patient's feelings of anger
  D. recognizing that the patient may feel hurt or discomfort
  E. setting strict limits

54. Bright light phototherapy is characterized by all of the following EXCEPT
  A. it increases melatonin in humans
  B. it requires exposure to the eyes of diffuse visible light
  C. it should be used daily
  D. treatments are given in the morning
  E. it is felt to help seasonal affective disorder

55. The treatment of neuroleptic malignant syndrome includes all of the following EXCEPT
   A. discontinuation of antipsychotic medications
   B. hot wraps to increase the core body temperature
   C. administration of dantrolene sodium (Dantrium)
   D. administration of bromocriptine (Parlodel)
   E. intravenous fluids

56. Placebo response is a well-recognized phenomenon in antidepressant trials. Which of the following factors generally predicts an increased placebo response rate?
   A. the presence of a full neurovegetative syndrome of depression
   B. more severe neurovegetative symptoms
   C. premorbid neurotic personality traits
   D. positive biological markers
   E. current episode greater than three months' duration

57. All of the following are effective agents for the treatment of attention-deficit hyperactivity disorder in children EXCEPT
   A. pemoline
   B. dextroamphetamine
   C. benztropine
   D. methylphenidate
   E. methamphetamine

58. Outpatient group psychotherapy is commonly NOT beneficial for patients diagnosed as having
   A. schizophrenia
   B. a major depressive episode
   C. antisocial personality disorder
   D. posttraumatic stress disorder
   E. alcohol dependence

59. The MOST widely used psychoactive drug in the world is
   A. diazepam
   B. caffeine
   C. nicotine
   D. alcohol
   E. cocaine

60. A patient who drinks alcohol while taking disulfiram (Antabuse) is likely to experience all of the following EXCEPT
  A. tachycardia
  B. vomiting
  C. sedation
  D. flushing
  E. hypotension

61. Brief psychotherapy is contraindicated for a patient who has
  A. sleep-onset insomnia
  B. dysphoric mood
  C. a psychosis
  D. marital problems
  E. a social phobia

DIRECTIONS (Questions 62 through 66): For each sexual dysfunction described in the questions below, select the appropriate behavioral intervention in headings A through E. Each heading may be used once, more than once, or not at all.

  A. gradual dilation of the vaginal opening with fingers
  B. "squeeze" technique
  C. creation of a nondemanding sexual situation
  D. masturbatory exercises
  E. stimulation of penis in close proximity to the vaginal opening

62. Premature ejaculation

63. Vaginismus

64. Primary anorgasmia in females

65. Ejaculatory incompetence

66. Impotence

DIRECTIONS (Questions 67 through 100): Each group of questions below consists of lettered headings followed by a list of numbered words, phrases, or statements. For each numbered word, phrase, or statement, select the ONE lettered heading that is most closely associated with it. Each lettered heading may be selected once, more than once, or not at all.

Questions 67 through 71:

    A. positive reinforcement
    B. escape conditioning
    C. extinction
    D. reciprocal inhibition
    E. flooding

67. Substitution of a favorable response for an unwanted behavior

68. Habit weakening through the elimination of any reward

69. Exposing patients to strongly anxiety-arousing stimuli

70. Response rendered more probable if followed by a reward

71. Removal of noxious stimulus constitutes the reward

Questions 72 through 75

    A. confrontation
    B. clarification
    C. interpretation
    D. empathic validation
    E. dream analysis

72. Allowing the patient to feel that his/her therapist understands his/her subjective experience

73. Making conscious the unconscious origins of the patient's observable behavior

74. Making explicit the details of behavioral patterns, character traits, resistances, and transferential attitudes

75. Highlighting aspects of behavior that must be faced by the patient

Questions 76 through 80

    A. increase in sleep latency
    B. increase in REM sleep
    C. decrease in REM sleep
    D. causes cataplexy

76. Alcohol

77. Reserpine

78. Caffeine

79. MAOI

80. Benzodiazepines

Questions 81 through 85

    A. fluoxetine
    B. desipramine
    C. amphetamine
    D. haloperidol
    E. monoamine oxidase inhibitor

81. Blocks catabolism of neurotransmitter

82. Inhibits reuptake of norepinephrine primarily

83. Inhibits reuptake of serotonin primarily

84. Releases CNS dopamine stores

85. Dangerous in combination with tyramine

Questions 86 through 90

    A. high potency
    B. low potency
    C. reliable IM absorption
    D. no physiologic dependence
    E. shortest half-life

86. Clonazepam

87. Midazolam

88. Lorazepam

89. Halazepam

90. Buspirone

Questions 91 through 95

    A. antiserotonergic 5HT2
    B. antiD2 dopaminergic
    C. GABA
    D. noradrenergic
    E. serotonergic

91. Maprotiline

92. Fluphenazine

93. Fluoxetine

94. Clozapine

95. Quazepam

Questions 96 through 100

    A. lithium
    B. alprazolam
    C. nortriptyline
    D. propranolol
    E. carbamazepine

96. Can cause leukocytosis

97. Lowers seizure threshold

98. Can cause leukopenia

99. Can cause severe withdrawal

100. Can lead to an asthma attack

Treatment

Explanatory Answers

1. (B) The mechanism of action of antipsychotic agents is the blockade of CNS dopaminergic receptors. All standard antipsychotic agents available in the United States, except for clozapine, are strong D2 dopamine receptor antagonists. (**Ref. 10,** pp. 97–99)

2. (B) Tacrine raises the level of acetylcholine in the synaptic cleft. It may delay or temporarily decrease the cognitive deficits seen in Alzheimer's disease. (**Ref. 1,** p. 985)

3. (E) Anticholinergic side effects include: dry mouth, blurred vision, tachycardia, urinary retention, and constipation. They can occur at therapeutic doses of many psychiatric medications, especially the tricyclic antidepressants. Severe anticholinergic toxicity leads to CNS impairment—difficulty with immediate recall, agitation, delirium, and visual hallucinations. Olfactory hallucinations can be a symptom of temporal lobe epilepsy. (**Ref. 1,** p. 898)

4. (C) Tardive dyskinesia typically consists of grimacing and buccofacial–mandibular movements. It can include choreiform and jerky movements of the arms, fingers, legs, and toes. It is thought that long-term blockade of dopamine receptors produces a degenerative hypersensitivity, with the formation of an increased number of receptor sites. It is a long-term side effect. (**Ref. 10,** pp. 167, 229)

5. (D) Most clinicians will look for at least a mild response at two to three weeks and then wait until at least four to six weeks at the therapeutic dose before stopping the trial. In some patients, the full response can take longer to be realized. (**Ref. 10,** p. 223)

6. (E) While hallucinations can occur with or without a delirium, frank delusions are not expected. Seizures can also occur after abrupt discontinuation of any benzodiazepine but have been most often reported with alprazolam. (**Ref. 10,** p. 436)

7. (B) Reducing the dose of the antidepressant medication in the maintenance period leads to increased recurrence of depression. After three episodes the risk of recurrence increases to over 90%. (**Ref. 10,** pp. 224–225)

8. (B) Sertraline may mildly inhibit the P-450 system but does not cause dramatic increases in other drug blood levels as Prozac can. Fluoxetine has a long half-life and an active metabolite with an even longer half-life. (**Ref. 10,** pp. 232, 245, 262)

9. (D) Seizures more often occur with levels above 2.5 to 3.0 mEq/L, along with coma, choreoathetosis and spontaneous attacks of hyperextension of the extremities. Other **early** signs include dysarthria and lack of coordination. (**Ref. 10,** p. 397)

10. (C) Most patients respond to blood levels in the 0–8 to 1–2 mEq/L range and will maintain at that level. Some patients who have not fully responded may benefit from and tolerate blood levels in the 1–2 to 1–5 mEq/L range. (**Ref. 10,** p. 354)

11. (D) NMS can best be thought of as a hypodopaminergic, hyperpyrexia syndrome induced by a wide range of dopamine blocking agents, not just antipsychotics. The majority of the cases occur in the first few weeks of medication initiation or dosage increase. (**Ref. 10,** p. 170)

12. (C) There is no evidence that valproic acid is an effective antipsychotic. It is an effective antiseizure agent that has found multiple alternative indication in psychiatry. (**Ref. 10,** pp. 383, 438, 458)

13. (**A**) Lithium has a myriad of clinical side effects that also includes muscle weakness, nausea, diarrhea and tremor. Polydipsia and polyuria occur in 60% of lithium patients. (**Ref. 10,** p. 393)

14. (**C**) In older patients or patients with a history of cardiac problems a prelithium electrocardiogram is recommended. As verapamil is often used in patients with cardiac disease, care must be taken in using it on patients taking lithium because it lowers the blood level of lithium. (**Ref. 10,** p. 394)

15. (**A**) Naloxone is a narcotic antagonist. Its use produces a withdrawal syndrome in patients addicted to opiates. (**Ref. 1,** pp. 445, 446)

16. (**D**) The presence of an intracranial mass is the only absolute contraindication to ECT because of the sudden increase in intracranial pressure during the procedure. Some patients with small intracranial masses can still be given ECT if pretreated with dexamethasone and if the intraseizure rise in blood pressure is controlled. (**Ref. 1,** p. 1010)

17. (**E**) All antipsychotic agents can cross the placenta. Antipsychotics can also be secreted in the mother's milk. The risk of birth defects with exposure to antipsychotics is not clear at this time. (**Ref. 1,** p. 872)

18. (**D**) Multiple types of data are used in biofeedback. The particular type of biofeedback used is matched to the patient's dominant pattern of psychophysiologic reactivity. The DST has no bearing on biofeedback. (**Ref. 1,** pp. 850, 851)

19. (**B**) Benzodiazepines promote the attachment of GABA to the GABA-a recognition site, which leads to enhancing GABA's inhibitory effects. There are few drug–drug interactions to worry about—the direct effects are the most problematic. (**Ref. 10,** pp. 415, 432)

20. (A) In operant conditioning, learning occurs as a result of the consequences of one's actions and their effect upon the environment. It is in classical conditioning that the animal is passive or restrained. (**Ref. 1,** p. 166)

21. (E) Countertransference refers to the therapist's relating to the patient as to someone from his own past (that is, his transference) or his responses to the patient's transference. (**Ref. 2,** p. 1448)

22. (A) Although tricyclic coma is short, it may result in death due to cardiac bradyarrhythmias. Tricyclic myocardial depressant and quinidine-like effects are important in this phenomenon. Patients in tricyclic coma should be monitored in a cardiac inpatient unit. (**Ref. 2,** p. 1647)

23. (D) Crisis intervention deals with people in the midst of a crisis in which rapid treatment is essential. It can utilize multiple techniques to treat the issue at hand. Personality change is a goal of long term psychotherapy and psychoanalysis. (**Ref. 1,** pp. 836–837)

24. (A) At best, clozapine may be effective for 30% of standard antipsychotic nonresponders. Although it causes significantly less extrapyramidal symptoms, it is not without significant side effects. (**Ref. 10,** pp. 108, 168, 178)

25. (A) Anti-parkinsonian drugs are used in the treatment of the extrapyramidal (motor) side effects of haloperidol and other antipsychotic agents. Use of parenteral agents can be helpful to differentiate exacerbation of psychosis from acute extrapyramidal side effects because they can work in minutes. (**Ref. 10,** p. 165)

26. (C) Suicide occurs more often in men. In contrast to the population as a whole, the greatest age at risk for suicide is shifted to the middle-aged in psychiatric patients. Psychiatric patients are estimated to have an incidence of self injury 50 times greater than the general population. (**Ref. 1,** p. 808; **Ref. 10,** p. 203)

27. (B) Standard antipsychotics can cause elevated prolactin levels leading to breast enlargement and lactation while thioridazine may lead to delayed ejaculation. Although antipsychotics may shift the glucose-tolerance curve in a diabetic fashion, frank diabetes mellitus has not been reported. (**Ref. 10,** p. 176)

28. **(E)**   Acute overdose of a tricyclic antidepressant results in anticholinergic symptoms, CNS toxicity, and possible cardiovascular collapse. (**Ref. 2,** p. 1644)

29. **(C)**   Surprisingly, acute psychotic patients judged as much improved or in remission had a pooled placebo response rate of 12% versus 45% for active treatment. Parenteral preparations avoid a first-pass effect and so are more bioavailable. (**Ref. 10,** pp. 103–115)

30. **(B)**   While propranolol may help reduce aggression in a patient population with congenital or acquired brain damage, there is no convincing evidence it is useful for antisocial personality disorder. Many consider it the treatment of choice for akathisia. (**Ref. 10,** pp. 165, 277, 395, 497)

31. **(E)**   Most antipsychotics can lower seizure threshhold, but it is rarely a clinically significant problem. Answers A, B, and D may be caused by chlorpromazine. Thioridazine may cause retinitis pigmentosa in doses above 800 mg per day. (**Ref. 10,** pp. 169–178)

32. **(C)**   Panic attacks can be effectively treated with benzodiazepines (especially alprazolam), monoamine oxidase inhibitors, and tricyclic antidepressants (especially imipramine). Cognitive behavioral therapy is useful in mastering the fear of recurrent attacks in specific phobic situations. Lithium is the drug of choice for bipolar disorder. (**Ref. 2,** p. 1584)

33. **(A)**   Pimozide, a high-potency antipsychotic, is effective in the treatment of monosymptomatic hypochondriasis. (**Ref. 1,** p. 1027)

34. **(E)**   Lithium use in psychiatric practice has gone beyond the treatment of bipolar disease. Other indications include the treatment of cyclothymia, schizoaffective disorder, and the potentiation of tricyclic antidepressants, but it has not been shown useful in schizophrenia. (**Ref. 1,** p. 926; **Ref. 2,** pp. 1637, 1657, 1658)

35. (B) A variety of psychiatric uses of beta-blocking agents have been reported in the literature. These include the treatment of performance anxiety, neuroleptic-induced akathisia, lithium tremor, and impulse control problems in patients with organic brain syndromes, but not tardive dyskinesia. (**Ref. 1,** p. 983; **Ref. 2,** pp. 1613, 1660, 1877)

36. (C) Obsessive–compulsive disorder is most effectively treated with a combination of serotonin reuptake blockers (clomipramine or fluoxetine) and behavior therapy (exposure and response prevention). (**Ref. 1,** p. 998)

37. (A) Psychostimulants (dextroamphetamine, methamphetamine, methylphenidate, and pemoline) were reclassified by the FDA in 1970 to the most restrictive classification for drugs that are medically useful (schedule II). They currently are approved for treatment of attention-deficit hyperactivity and narcolepsy. Psychiatric uses include treatment of severe depression in specific patient populations and pain management. Appetite suppression is *not* an indication for the use of these medications. (**Ref. 2,** pp. 1184, 1251)

38. (D) The most successful behavioral interventions in the treatment of obesity include: increasing awareness of eating behaviors through self-monitoring techniques, developing control over stimuli that precede eating behavior, limiting availability of high-calorie foods in the home setting, and confining all eating to one place. (**Ref. 2,** p. 1183)

39. (B) Wernicke's encephalopathy is an acute life-threatening complication of chronic alcohol use. Thiamine deficiency secondary to a prolonged inadequate diet is thought to be the causative factor. Immediate thiamine replacement is indicated. (**Ref. 2,** p. 1441)

40. (E) Hypnosis is a technique, *not* a form of therapy. It is most effective when integrated into an ongoing psychotherapeutic process. (**Ref. 2,** p. 1509)

41. (B) It is not cross-tolerant with any sedative hypnotic, including alcohol. Onset of action is similar to antidepressants and can take one to two weeks. (**Ref. 10,** p. 420)

42. (B) Of patients with a severe major depressive episode with melancholia, 80% to 90% will have a satisfactory response to ECT. Depressed patients with psychotic features also have a more favorable response to ECT as compared to antidepressant medications by themselves. (**Ref. 2,** p. 1676)

43. (A) Presently, there is research supporting only the use of antidepressants in the pharmacologic treatment of bulimia nervosa. (**Ref. 2,** p. 1862)

44. (E) Management of the violent patient includes seclusion, restraint (if necessary), medical evaluation, and possible pharmacologic treatment (beta-blocking agents, lithium, or carbamazepine). (**Ref. 2,** p. 1429)

45. (A) The *amount* of GI absorption is not significantly altered by the aging process; however, the *rate* of absorption may be lowered. (**Ref. 2,** p. 2039)

46. (E) Depressive symptoms most likely to respond to antidepressive medications are the vegetative ones—appetite and sleep disturbances, decreased energy, decreased libido, diurnal mood variation, and psychomotor retardation. Symptoms less likely to respond are those that are more subjective and psychological in nature—demoralization, low self-esteem, hopelessness, and helplessness. (**Ref. 1,** p. 896)

47. (E) All candidates for psychosurgery must have an intractable and devastating condition unrelieved by other therapies. (**Ref. 2,** p. 1678)

48. (E) Systematic desensitization involves approaching anxiety-provoking situations in a gradual and relaxed state of mind. Visual imagery is initially utilized, followed by "in vivo" challenges. Implosion, on the other hand, requires confrontation of a feared situation through imagery at *full intensity* for a prolonged period, until it is no longer frightening. (**Ref. 1,** p. 263)

49. (D) Cognitive therapy is a model of short-term psychotherapy, initially developed for the treatment of depression and anxiety. It is based on the premise that emotional dysfunction is caused by patients' distorted and often irrational views of themselves and the world. (**Ref. 2,** p. 1541)

50. (B) Structural family therapy focuses on the different roles and interactions occurring among family members, especially between generations. Intervention techniques involve realigning boundaries and alliances. (**Ref. 2,** p. 1540)

51. (A) Panic-prone individuals, as compared to normal subjects, are more likely to experience a panic attack following the administration of lactate IV, yohimbine, carbon dioxide, caffeine, and isoproterenol. These may be used as diagnostic tests. (**Ref. 1,** p. 699)

52. (C) Therapeutic effect requires plasma levels of 6.0 to 12.0 mg/L. The usual daily dose range of carbamazepine is 600 to 1200 mg per day, administered in divided doses. (**Ref. 2,** p. 1681)

53. (E) Behind anger there is usually hurt. Frequently, the angry person feels discounted—his expectations or needs are not being met. Consequently, it is necessary first to listen. Sometimes it is sufficient for the patient to ventilate. At times, an apology is appropriate. Compromise may be indicated. An important way of obtaining patient compliance is simply to ask if the treatment plan is agreeable and, if not, what needs to be included. (**Ref. 1,** p. 144)

54. (A) Bright light phototherapy decreases melatonin production in humans. Although considered experimental at this point in time, it may help with circadian disruptions, such as jet lag, delayed sleep syndrome, and chronobiologic disorders in shift workers. (**Ref. 10,** pp. 319–323)

55. (E) Neuroleptic malignant syndrome (NMS) is a medical emergency requiring intensive medical support. Cooling blankets and ice packs are needed at times to lower the core body temperature of the patient. (**Ref. 10,** p. 172)

56. (C) Day-to-day mood fluctuations, reactive mood, and premorbid neurotic personality traits positively correlate with a placebo effect. Melancholic symptoms have a lower placebo response. (**Ref. 10,** p. 223)

57. **(C)** Attention-deficit hyperactivity disorder in children is pharmacologically treated with CNS stimulants, which include dextroamphetamine, methamphetamine, methylphenidate, and pemoline. **(Ref. 2,** p. 1835)

58. **(C)** Antisocial persons, in general, tend to be resistant to all forms of psychotherapy. Their inability to feel loyalty and maintain confidentiality make them particularly unsuited for group experiences. **(Ref. 2,** p. 1524)

59. **(B)** Of adult Americans, 20% to 30% consume greater that 500 mg of caffeine per day. **(Ref. 1,** p. 683)

60. **(C)** Disulfiram blocks the normal oxidation of alcohol, causing acetaldehyde accumulation in the bloodstream. Acetaldehyde is highly toxic and produces nausea, vomiting, hypotension, tachycardia, and flushing. **(Ref. 1,** p. 698)

61. **(C)** Brief psychotherapy is best suited for patients with fairly well-circumscribed problems but who are otherwise functioning well psychologically. The presence of psychotic symptoms indicates a serious, more pervasive psychiatric problem that usually requires pharmacotherapy. **(Ref. 2,** p. 1564)

62. **(B)** Premature ejaculation is the chief complaint of 35% to 40% of men treated for sexual disorders. The squeeze technique involves the firm application of pressure on the coronal ridge of the penis at the point of impending orgasm, thus preventing ejaculation. **(Ref. 1,** p. 666)

63. **(A)** Vaginismus most often afflicts women who are highly educated and those in high socioeconomic groups. Vaginismus describes the involuntary spasm of vaginal musculature, which prevents penetration. It can be treated with gentle dilation of the vaginal opening using fingers or mechanical dilators. This exercise is repeated until the man is able to insert his penis into the vagina without discomfort to his female partner. **(Ref. 1,** p. 667)

64. **(D)** Anorgasmia is found in only 5% of married women over the age of 35 years. It may respond to masturbatory techniques,

including, in some cases, the use of a mechanical vibrator. (**Ref. 1,** pp. 664, 665)

65. (**E**)   Ejaculatory incompetence is also known as male orgasmic disorder, in which the man cannot ejaculate during coitus. Treatment strategies include the stimulation of the penis in close proximity to the vaginal opening, followed by quick insertion into the vagina at the point of orgasm and ejaculation. (**Ref. 1,** p. 665)

66. (**C**)   Impotence is the chief complaint in more than 50% of men treated for sexual disorders. If the impotence is nonorganic in nature, a low-anxiety sexual situation that allows the man to achieve an erection without the pressure of intercourse may help. (**Ref. 1,** p. 664)

67. (**D**)   In using systematic desensitization, a patient is helped to attain a completely relaxed state and then is exposed to a phobic stimulus that typically causes anxiety in the patient. The patient's anxiety is then inhibited because he/she is in a relaxed state. This process is call reciprocal inhibition. (**Ref. 10,** p. 852)

68. (**C**)   In classical (Pavlovian) conditioning an unconditioned stimulus (food) that will elicit an unconditioned response (salivating in dogs) is paired with a conditioned stimulus (a bell being struck). With repetition, the conditioned stimulus alone will elicit the unconditioned response. If the conditioned stimulus is continuously presented without the unconditioned stimulus, the unconditioned response will no longer occur. This is known as extinction. (**Ref. 10,** p. 166)

69. (**E**)   It is thought by some that when a patient escapes from an adversive/phobic situation that causes anxiety for him/her that if he/she do this repetitively it reinforces his/her anxiety through conditioning. Flooding encourages the patient to confront the anxiety-provoking stimulus directly and suddenly without relaxation techniques or gradual exposure. The patient remains in contact with the stimulus until his/her anxiety subsides. (**Ref. 10,** p. 854)

70. (**A**)   Token economies are an example of positive reinforcement. If any behavioral response (good or bad) is followed by a reward

(eg, money, food), it tends to become strengthened and increase in frequency. (**Ref. 10,** p. 855)

71. (B) Escape conditioning is a type of negative reinforcement. If an animal is placed in a situation wherein it will experience an adversive event (eg, a shock through the cage bottom), it will reinforce behaviors that lessen the likelihood of experiencing the adversive event again (jumping off the cage bottom). The escape behavior will increase in frequency. (**Ref. 10,** p. 167)

72. (D) Empathic validation is an intervention that shows the patient that the therapist is in tune with his/her feelings. When this occurs, it is thought to increase the patient's ability to accept the therapist's interpretations. (**Ref. 10,** p. 829)

73. (C) Interpretation connects thoughts, feelings, and behaviors of current life with those in the patient's unconscious. It is the hallmark therapeutic instrument in insight-oriented treatments (**Ref. 10,** p. 829)

74. (B) Clarification is separating unimportant aspects of therapeutic material from the important aspects that help the patient articulate something he/she is having difficulty conveying. Clarification differs from confrontation because it does not involve the patient who is presenting with denial or minimization. (**Ref. 10,** p. 829)

75. (A) Confrontation addresses therapeutic material that the patient does not want to address or is minimizing or avoiding. Confrontation need not be experienced as harsh and can lead the patient to discuss important issues. (**Ref. 10,** p. 829)

76. (C) Alcohol may ease entry into sleep for some but has negative effects on sleep architecture. It decreases REM and deep (stage 4) sleep, and increases sleep fragmentation. (**Ref. 1,** p. 401)

77. (B) Reserpine can increase REM sleep and cause depression. Antidepressants reduce REM sleep. (**Ref. 1,** p. 702)

78. (A) Caffeine intoxication can cause increased sleep latency, inability to remain asleep, and early morning awakening. It is notable that caffeine is a more potent methylxanthine than theophylline. (**Ref. 1,** pp. 416, 418)

79. **(C)** MAOI-treated patients have significantly decreased REM sleep. It can manifest in patients as daytime drowsiness secondary to nighttime insomnia. (**Ref. 1,** p. 972)

80. **(C)** All benzodiazepines lead to a moderate decrease in REM sleep but are not associated with REM rebound when stopped. Benzodiazepines also decrease stage 3 and stage 4 sleep. (**Ref. 1,** p. 910)

81. **(E)** Monoamine oxidase inhibitors (MAOI) prevent the breakdown (catabolism) of neurotransmitters, such as serotonin, norepinephrine, and dopamine. It is thought by most that inhibition of MAO is the primary antidepressant action of these medications. (**Ref. 10,** p. 972)

82. **(B)** Desipramine has more norepinephrine reuptake blockage effects than imipramine, amitriptyline, nortriptyline, clomipramine, and cloxepin. Among the secondary amine tricyclic antidepressants, desipramine also has the least anticholinergic activity. (**Ref. 10,** pp. 992, 995)

83. **(A)** The selective serotonin reuptake inhibitors (SSRIs) (fluoxetine, sertraline and paroxetine) all inhibit the reuptake of serotonin, which is thought to lead to their antidepressant effects. They lack clinically significant agonist or antagonist activities at anticholinergic, antihistaminergic, anti-alpha, and anti-adrenergic receptors and thus have a low incidence of side effects. (**Ref. 10,** p. 976)

84. **(C)** Amphetamine is a sympathomimetic that works by stimulating the release of dopamine from presynaptic terminals. The sympathomimetics are useful in treating depression in some special patient populations, such as the seriously medically ill, but this usefulness must be weighed against their abuse potential. (**Ref. 10,** p. 981)

85. **(E)** Patients on a nonselective MAOI may be at risk for a lethal hypertensive crisis secondary to MAOa inhibitor in the GI tract

that leads to increased tyramine absorption. The use of MAOI is also prohibited with multiple other drugs. These drugs include anesthetics with epinephrine, anti-asthma agents, antihypertensives, narcotics, L-dopa, over the counter and prescribed sympathomimetics, and SSRIs. (**Ref. 10,** pp. 974, 975)

86. **(A)** Clonazepam has high potency along with alprazolam, estazolam, and triazolam. It differs markedly from the other high-potency benzodiazepines in that it has a long half-life. (**Ref. 1,** p. 913)

87. **(E)** Midazolam has the shortest half-life of the benzodiazepines listed. Only triazolam has a similar half-life. Midazolam produces strong amnestic effects and is used in sedation for medical procedures. (**Ref. 1,** pp. 907, 908, 913)

88. **(C)** Ativan has a moderate absorption rate by mouth but is rapidly absorbed following intramuscular injection. The rapidity of its intramuscular absorption makes it an essential medication in the treatment of psychotic agitation in the emergency setting. (**Ref. 1,** p. 907, 910)

89. **(B)** Halazepam has a dosage range of 60 to 160 mg; it has the lowest potency of currently available antipsychotics and has a long half-life. Oxazepam is another low-potency benzodiazepine, but it has a short half-life. (**Ref. 1,** p. 913)

90. **(D)** Buspirone is chemically distinct from the benzodiazepines, does not directly affect GABA, and is not thought to cause physiological dependence. It also does not have sedative, hypnotic, muscle-relaxant, or anti-convulsant effects. (**Ref. 1,** p. 921)

91. **(D)** Maprotiline is a relatively selective norepinephrine reuptake blocker, as is desipramine. Maprotiline has relatively more seizure threshold lowering effect than the tricyclic antidepressants or the other tetracyclic amoxapines. (**Ref. 1,** pp. 992, 996)

92. **(B)** Fluphenazine shares in common with all current antipsychotics, except clozaril, the ability to antagonize D2 dopaminer-

gic receptor activity. The intensity of the antipsychotic effects of all current antipsychotics, except clozaril, is more correlated with their relative affinity at blocking D2 dopaminergic receptors. (**Ref. 1,** p. 994)

93. (**E**)   Fluoxetine is an antidepressant in the selective serotonin reuptake inhibitor (SSRI) class. It has minimal effects on other neurotransmitter symptoms. (**Ref. 1,** p. 976)

94. (**A**)   Clozapine has very low D2 dopaminergic receptor antagonism effects. It does exhibit antagonism at D1 dopaminergic, 5HT2 serotonergic, and alpha-1 noradrenergic receptors. It is considered an atypical antipsychotic because of its neurotransmitter effects, which are different than those seen in "typical" or "standard" antipsychotics. (**Ref. 1,** p. 933)

95. (**C**)   Quazepam is a benzodiazepine and increases GABA-a receptor affinity for GABA. Quazepam and halazepam are relatively more specific for BZ1 receptors than BZ2 receptors. As BZ2 receptors are believed to be more involved in cognition, memory, and motor control, quazepam and halazepam might be expected to cause less amnestic effects. (**Ref. 1,** p. 908)

96. (**A**)   Lithium counts among its many side effects leukocytosis, which is benign. (**Ref. 1,** p. 964)

97. (**C**)   Nortriptyline and other tricyclic and tetracyclic antidepressants all lower the seizure threshold to some extent. The SSRIs also appear to lower the seizure threshold comparable to the incidence seen with other antidepressants. (**Ref. 1,** pp. 978, 996)

98. (**E**)   Carbamazepine causes a benign suppression of white blood cells with severe blood dyscrasia 5 (aplastic anemia, agranulocytosis) occurring in about 1 of 20,000 patients taking it. Antipsychotics other than clozapine can also cause leukopenia, as well as mild anemia, and rarely agranulocytosis. (**Ref. 1,** pp. 285, 926)

99. **(B)** Alprazolam is a very high potency, short half-life benzodiazepine that can cause a sudden and severe withdrawal syndrome if stopped suddenly. It should be tapered off slowly before being discontinued. (**Ref. 1,** pp. 911, 912)

100. **(D)** Propranolol can precipitate an asthma attack, as well as hypotension and bradycardia. Its neuropsychiatric uses include treating social phobia, lithium-induced postural tremor, and neuroleptic-induced acute akathisia. (**Ref. 1,** pp. 893, 894)

7

Ethical and Legal Aspects of Psychiatry

Joseph B. Layde
John E. Pappenheim

DIRECTIONS (Questions 1 through 18): Each of the questions or incomplete statements below is followed by five suggested answers or completions. Select the ONE that is best in each case.

---

1. Which of the following is NOT used as a criterion for establishing testamentary capacity?
   A. knowing the nature and extent of one's property
   B. knowing the natural object of one's bounty
   C. knowing that one is making a will
   D. knowing the difference between right and wrong
   E. none of the above

2. A 50-year-old man has been scheduled for electroconvulsive therapy because his depression and suicidal behavior have not improved on psychotropic medication. The patient understands the risks and benefits of the treatment and refuses ECT. His attorney files a writ of habeas corpus. The major issue is
   A. the patient has a right to treatment
   B. the patient has a right to refuse treatment

    C. the psychiatrist must warn interested parties of the danger of the treatment

    D. the right of treatment is a corollary of deprivation of liberty

    E. ECT is a cruel and unusual punishment

3. A 55-year-old chronic schizophrenic patient who has been involuntarily hospitalized sues the hospital on the grounds that he is receiving no therapy. He has not had a documented physical examination or psychiatric evaluation for over a year. The counsel is likely to base his case on

    A. the constitutional right to refuse treatment

    B. the importance of informed consent prior to treatment

    C. res ipsa loquitur

    D. the right to treatment in return for confinement

    E. testamentary capacity

4. Which of the following statements is NOT true regarding psychiatric malpractice?

    A. there have been successful suits against psychiatrists for sexual exploitation of their patients in the context of psychiatric treatment

    B. most insurance companies indemnify psychiatrists against suits for sexual exploitation

    C. psychiatrists are now more willing and available to testify that their colleagues were negligent than in the past

    D. biological treatments with physical side effects can cause damages familiar to lawyers and judges

    E. the change in the practice of psychiatry to high-volume, short-term care, has made the doctor–patient relationship more impersonal

5. Competency to stand trial is

    A. criminal responsibility for one's conduct

    B. understanding the wrongfulness of one's act

    C. the ability to understand the legal proceedings one faces and to rationally consult with one's lawyer

    D. the ability to understand the side effects of medications

    E. irrelevant in modern American legal practice

6. Which of the following is NOT true regarding psychiatric testimony?

  A. a psychiatrist may be required to give testimony outside of court in the form of a deposition

  B. a psychiatrist must respond to a court subpoena to testify or face punishment as being in contempt of court

  C. psychiatrists may be qualified as expert witnesses to provide technical data and express their relevant opinions on psychiatric matters

  D. it is ethical for doctors to agree to testify for the plaintiff in a civil suit in return for a certain percentage of the plaintiff's recovery

  E. if a state allows the insanity defense, the U.S. constitution requires the state to provide funds for employment of a psychiatric expert for an indigent criminal defendant

7. The verdict of "guilty but mentally ill" is

  A. basically another name for the insanity defense

  B. a guarantee that an offender will receive treatment for mental illness

  C. a means of mitigating a person's criminal sentence

  D. used in some states alongside a traditional verdict of not guilty by reason of insanity

  E. endorsed by the American Psychiatric Association and the American Bar Association

8. To support a claim of negligence, all of the following are true EXCEPT

  A. a standard of care must exist

  B. a duty must be owed by the defendant or someone for whose conduct he is answerable

  C. there must be a breach of the duty owed to the plaintiff

  D. the plaintiff must be damaged by the defendant's actions

  E. the plaintiff must show the defendant acted with malevolence

9. The *M'Naughten* rule for the insanity defense states that a defendant must have been laboring under such a deficit of reason from disease of the mind at the time he committed a criminal act that

  A. he did not know the nature and quality of the act he was doing, or if he did know it, he did not know what he was doing was wrong

    B. he was unable to resist an impulse to commit an act

    C. his act was the product of mental disease

    D. he was suffering from auditory hallucinations at the time of the defense

    E. his behavior was like that of a "wild animal"

10. Which of the following is NOT a major source of law in the United States?

    A. state and federal statutes

    B. state and federal constitutions

    C. case law

    D. administrative rules

    E. unwritten criminal law

11. Involuntary drug treatment could be the basis of a civil suit based on all of the following EXCEPT

    A. a malpractice claim of battery

    B. negligent failure to provide informed consent

    C. a violation of a constitutional right to privacy

    D. the insanity defense

    E. a constitutional right to self-determination

12. Which of the following persons does NOT have a duty to raise the issue of a defendant's competency to stand trial if he/she believes that the defendant may be mentally ill and that such illness may interfere with the defendant's capacity to stand trial?

    A. district attorney

    B. defense psychiatrist

    C. prosecutor

    D. defense attorney

    E. judge

13. Psychiatric testimony frequently is required in each of the following legal cases EXCEPT

    A. actions for damages for emotional distress

    B. worker's compensation cases

    C. psychiatric malpractice cases

    D. free speech cases

    E. child custody cases

14. Under which of the following circumstances does the law require reporting of suspected child abuse by a psychiatrist who evaluates a child?
    A. in all cases
    B. only when the psychiatrist believes it is in the child's best interest
    C. only when consent of a parent or guardian is obtained
    D. only in cases in which the child shows behavioral manifestations of abuse
    E. only when the psychiatrist has examined all members of the family

15. Which of the following is a hallmark of the Anglo-American system of justice?
    A. the adversarial system
    B. the inquisitorial system
    C. the scientific method
    D. trial in absentia
    E. the Napoleonic code

16. In which state did the legal "duty to protect" third parties from dangerous outpatients arise?
    A. Alaska
    B. Arizona
    C. California
    D. Oregon
    E. Wisconsin

17. In what year was child abuse first reported as a clinical phenomenon?
    A. 1852
    B. 1891
    C. 1910
    D. 1945
    E. 1962

18. Which of the following is NOT considered a risk factor contributing to child abuse?
    A. parental personality traits
    B. vocational stress and unemployment of parents

C. normal intelligence of children
D. financial insecurity
E. intra-family dynamics

DIRECTIONS (Questions 19 through 32): Each group of questions below consists of lettered headings followed by a list of numbered words, phrases, or statements. For each numbered word, phrase, or statement, select the ONE lettered heading that is most closely associated with it. Each lettered heading may be selected once, more than once, or not at all.

Questions 19 and 20

A. *Durham* decision
B. *M'Naughten* rule

19. Judge David Bazelon

20. Attempted assassination of Sir Robert Peel

Questions 21 through 24

A. right to treatment
B. civil commitment
C. duty to warn third parties
D. testamentary capacity
E. criminal responsibility

21. *Tarasoff* v. *Regents of the University of California*

22. *Youngberg* v. *Romeo*

23. *Lessard* v. *Schmidt*

24. *Durham* v. *United States*

Questions 25 through 28

    A. cognitive defect
    B. product of disease
    C. diminished capacity
    D. competency to stand trial
    E. cognitive or volitional defect

25. *Durham* test of insanity

26. *M'Naughten* test of insanity

27. American Law Institute (ALI) test of insanity

28. "Twinkie defense"

Questions 29 through 32

    A. justifiable violation of confidentiality
    B. never justifiable violation of ethics
    C. justifiable involuntary medication
    D. justifiable psychiatric testimony based on secondhand information
    E. never justifiable judicial interference

29. Imminent risk of physical injury

30. Testamentary capacity

31. Duty to protect

32. Patient–therapist sex

Ethical and Legal Aspects of Psychiatry

Explanatory Answers

1. **(D)** Testamentary capacity refers to the capacity to make a will. A valid will can be written by a person who knows what he is doing, knows what he owns, and knows who will benefit from the will and his relationship to those persons. (**Ref. 5,** pp. 820–821)

2. **(B)** The issues involved center around the competency of the mentally ill and the right to refuse treatment. It would seem, from the history, that this patient is competent to make decisions about his treatment, although he is very depressed. For consent to a therapy or medical procedure to be valid, it must be competent, knowing, and voluntary. (**Ref. 5,** pp. 817–819)

3. **(D)** The right to treatment has been formulated as an important legal question in all categories of noncriminal confinement. *Youngberg* v. *Romeo* is a recent applicable case. To fulfill this treatment right, a state must provide a humane physical and psychological environment, qualified staff in sufficient numbers, and individual treatment or rehabilitation plans for each patient. (**Ref. 5,** pp. 815–817)

4. **(B)** The rise of feminism made claims of sexual exploitation more credible in court, and more of such cases made their way

into the malpractice arena. Most insurers are no longer willing to indemnify psychiatrists against sexual misbehavior with their patients. (**Ref. 5,** pp. 821–822)

5. **(C)**   Incompetency to stand trial means a failure to rationally participate in the legal system. Criminal insanity, on the other hand, involves one's understanding of one's criminal behavior. (**Ref. 5,** pp. 806–808)

6. **(D)**   Contingency fee arrangements for testimony are unethical. The 1985 U.S. Supreme Count ruling in *Ake* v. *Oklahoma* held that states that allow the insanity defense must provide funds for the hiring of an indigent defendant's psychiatric expert. (**Ref. 2,** pp. 461–462)

7. **(D)**   The verdict of "guilty but mentally ill" is a new verdict used in several states that acknowledges the mental illness of a criminal wrongdoer, but neither mitigates a sentence nor mandates treatment for mental illness. The American Psychiatric Association and the American Bar Association have gone on record as opposed to the verdict of "guilty but mentally ill." (**Ref. 2,** p. 464)

8. **(E)**   Psychiatric malpractice is based on the negligence standard of law. That standard requires that a plaintiff's damages must be directly caused by a dereliction of a duty owed him by the defendant. (**Ref. 5,** pp. 821–823)

9. **(A)**   The *M'Naughten* test is followed in many U.S. jurisdictions. It concentrates on a knowledge of wrongfulness of his action on the part of a criminal defendant. (**Ref. 5,** pp. 803–805)

10. **(E)**   Law pertaining to psychiatry, as is the case with all areas of law, may come in the form of legislative decisions, court opinions, rules made by legal authorities, or constitutions. However, since it is important for people to know what is illegal so that they may avoid such acts, unwritten criminal law is not a source of law in the United States. (**Ref. 5,** pp. 799–802)

11. **(D)** Malpractice claims for involuntary drug treatment have become more common in recent years. The insanity defense applies solely to criminal law. **(Ref. 5, p. 798)**

12. **(B)** A psychiatrist does not have the obligation spelled out to court officers in *Pate* v. *Robinson* to question a defendant's competency to stand trial when it should be an issue. The district attorney and prosecutor are two names for the same official. **(Ref. 5, pp. 806–807)**

13. **(D)** Psychiatrists testify in many types of cases in the United States today. Free speech, however, is a constitutional issue, and one which would rarely involve psychiatric testimony. **(Ref. 2, pp. 468–469)**

14. **(A)** Clinicians are required to report all cases of suspected abuse of children they see in all jurisdictions in the United States. The law does not leave the issue to a clinician's discretion. **(Ref. 5, p. 631)**

15. **(A)** Judicial systems in much of Europe and much of the rest of the world actively involve the judge in ascertaining the facts, which is an inquisitorial system. The Napoleonic code is still the basis for most French law. In Britain and in the United States, on the other hand, the adversarial nature of judicial proceedings is paramount. The judge is impartial and waits for the respective attorneys to present evidence. **(Ref. 5, p. 801)**

16. **(C)** The California Supreme Court developed the doctrine that psychotherapists have a duty to protect identifiable third parties from the acts of their dangerous patients. The doctrine appears in the court's second opinion in the important case *Tarasoff v. Regents of the University of California,* written in 1976. **(Ref. 5, p. 823)**

17. **(E)** The classic paper, "The Battered Child Syndrome," by Kempe and co-workers, was published in 1962. It was the first report of child abuse as a clinical phenomenon. **(Ref. 2, p. 357)**

18. **(C)** Child abuse is related to parental personalities, parental unemployment and financial insecurity, and to poor family interdy-

namics. Mentally retarded and physically handicapped children are considered to be at higher risk for being abused than are normally developing children. (**Ref. 1,** pp. 786–787)

19. **(A)** In the 1954 *Durham* case, Judge David Bazelon ruled that "an accused is not criminally responsible if his unlawful act was the product of mental disease or mental defect." The *Durham* decision is no longer followed in the District of Columbia, where it originated. (**Ref. 2,** pp. 463–464)

20. **(B)** The 1843 *M'Naughten* rule came about after Daniel M'Naughten attempted to shoot British Prime Minister Sir Robert Peel. It makes the accused not criminally responsible for an act if he did not understand the nature and quality of his act and whether it was right or wrong. (**Ref. 5,** p. 803)

21. **(C)** *Tarasoff* v. *Regents of the University of California* first established the duty to warn and then to protect identifiable third parties from therapists' dangerous patients. It has been followed in many other states. (**Ref. 5,** p. 823)

22. **(A)** In *Youngberg* v. *Romeo,* the U.S. Supreme Court ruled that institutionalized mentally retarded patients have at least a narrow right to treatment. They have a right to a safe environment and to training necessary for their safety and freedom of movement. (**Ref. 5,** p. 816)

23. **(B)** *Lessard* v. *Schmidt,* a federal case arising in Wisconsin, set the trend for much more stringent requirements for the civil comment for psychiatric patients in the 1970s. Most states followed the trend to rewrite their commitment laws with more regard for patients' liberty interests. (**Ref. 5,** pp. 800, 814)

24. **(E)** *Durham* v. *United States* stated that a defendant was insane and not criminally responsible if his unlawful act was the product of mental disease or mental defect. It is no longer the law in any jurisdiction in the United States except the U.S. Virgin Islands. (**Ref. 2,** pp. 463–464)

25. **(B)** In 1954, Judge David Bazelon wrote the *Durham* decision. It held that a defendant could be found not criminally responsible

if his criminal act was the product of mental disease. (**Ref. 2,** pp. 463–464)

26. (**A**)   The *M'Naughten* test of insanity focuses specifically on the cognitive question of what a defendant believed about the rightness or wrongness of his act. It does not consider his ability to conform his conduct to the law. (**Ref. 5,** p. 803)

27. (**E**)   The American Law Institute test of insanity allows acquittal of a defendant under the insanity defense if the person "lacks substantial capacity either to appreciate the criminality of his conduct or to conform his conduct to the requirements of the law," as a result of mental disease or defect. This test considers both cognitive and volitional aspects of the defendant's capacity. (**Ref. 5,** pp. 804, 806)

28. (**C**)   California abolished the controversial doctrine of "diminished capacity" after Dan White, the killer of the mayor of San Francisco and another noted city official, successfully had his crime reduced from murder to manslaughter after his attorney argued that Mr. White was depressed and that his compulsive eating of junk foods was one symptom of that depression. The notion of diminished capacity was that a person might be guilty of a lesser crime if he has a mitigating mental disorder. (**Ref. 5,** p. 806)

29. (**C**)   Where there is imminent risk of physical injury by a patient to himself or to others, emergency medication may be involuntarily given to the patient. The medication may not continue to be involuntarily given once the emergency has passed, except by court order or a similar provision. (**Ref. 5,** p. 819)

30. (**D**)   Psychiatric ethics generally forbid the diagnosis of an individual whom a psychiatrist has not personally examined. However, when a person's testamentary capacity (capacity to write a will) is contested after a person's death, a psychiatrist is permitted to testify about an individual's apparent mental state as inferred from sources compiled while the individual was alive, eg, hospital records or letters. (**Ref. 5,** pp. 820–821)

31. (A)   The *Tarasoff* duty to protect identifiable third-party victims from a patient's dangerous behavior may require the treating psychiatrist to inform the threatened individual or legal authorities of the patient's threats. This can justify violating confidentiality. (**Ref. 5,** p. 823)

32. (B)   Patient–therapist sex is sexual exploitation and is malpractice. In some jurisdictions, it is also a felony. (**Ref. 5,** pp. 22–26, 822)

8

Case Studies

DIRECTIONS (Questions 1 through 60): This section consists of clinical situations, each followed by a series of questions. Study each situation and select the ONE best answer to each question following it.

Questions 1 through 3

A 38-year-old black woman comes to the emergency department of a general hospital with her husband. She is agitated, diaphoretic, and tremulous. She cries out in fear of visual hallucinations, saying, "Police are around that corner; they are trying to shoot me!" She has a history of one myocardial infarction and 20 years of insulin-dependent diabetes mellitus.

1. All of the following are important questions to ask the patient and her husband in the immediate evaluation of this patient EXCEPT
   - A. what food had the patient eaten in the 24 hours prior to presentation
   - B. what alcohol had the patient consumed in the past week
   - C. what were the timing and dosage of her insulin shots over the two days prior to presentation
   - D. does she have a history of similar episodes
   - E. does she suffer from phantom-limb syndrome

2. The MOST important single diagnostic test in this woman's immediate evaluation is
   A. a STAT glucose level
   B. serum TSH
   C. CT scan of the head
   D. electrocardiogram
   E. electroencephalogram

3. The MOST important immediate medication for this patient would include
   A. intramuscular lorazepam
   B. oral or intravenous glucose
   C. intramuscular haloperidol
   D. oral amoxapine
   E. oral fluoxetine

Questions 4 through 7

A 30-year-old white stockbroker comes to your office speaking rapidly and reporting that he has not been sleeping for the last week but feels very energetic. He states that he believes he has learned the ultimate secret to ensure making a killing on the stock market.

4. All of the following are important questions to ask this patient in your initial evaluation EXCEPT
   A. has he noticed a recent change in sexual desire
   B. does he have a history of appendectomy
   C. does he have a history of similar episodes
   D. has he recently engaged in reckless spending
   E. does he experience auditory hallucinations

5. Medication that is likely to give some relief of manic symptoms in this patient in a matter of hours rather than days includes
   A. lithium carbonate
   B. valproic acid
   C. haloperidol
   D. carbamazepine
   E. amitriptyline

6. Two weeks after his initial presentation, this stockbroker has achieved control of his manic episode on lithium carbonate. What is the therapeutic level of lithium for most acute manic episodes?
   A. 0.1 to 0.3 mEq/L
   B. 0.4 to 0.6 mEq/L
   C. 1.0 to 1.5 mEq/L
   D. 1.6 to 2.0 mEq/L
   E. 3.0 to 5.0 mEq/L

7. Long-term therapy of this man with lithium carbonate might be expected to leave him at increased risk of each of the following problems EXCEPT
   A. a decrease in the urine-concentrating ability of the kidneys
   B. decreased creatinine clearance by the kidneys
   C. a decrease in thyroid function
   D. malignant transformation of a skin nevus (mole)
   E. a fine tremor of the hands

Questions 8 through 10

A 25-year-old white woman presents to the emergency room of a general hospital after slightly cutting her arms with a razor blade during an argument with her boyfriend. She has a history of intense relationships, many of which have been short-lived, and a history of similar attempts at self-abuse at times of trouble in those relationships.

8. The single MOST important question to ask in the initial assessment of this patient is
   A. is there a history of sexual abuse of the patient
   B. is the patient suicidal or homicidal
   C. does the patient possess a cherished "transitional object," such as a teddy bear
   D. is the patient concerned about her sexual orientation
   E. has the patient been engaging in unsafe sexual practices

9. If this patient is admitted to an inpatient psychiatric ward, all of the following behaviors are likely to be seen EXCEPT

    A. the playing off one caregiver against another about management of the patient

    B. sexual acting out by the patient

    C. self-abusive behavior by the patient

    D. involuntary urinary incontinence by the patient

    E. alternate overvaluation and undervaluation of caregivers

10. Which of the following is the most likely long-term prognosis for such a patient with borderline personality disorder?

    A. a progression towards schizophrenia

    B. deterioration of relationships and vocational functioning in her 30s and 40s

    C. little risk of episodes of major depressive disorder

    D. increasing stability in relationships and vocational functioning during midlife

    E. little risk of self-harm

Questions 11 through 13

A 50-year-old divorced woman presents for psychiatric evaluation in January 1994. She complains of depressed mood since October 1993, becoming progressively worse. In addition, she complains of tearfulness, impaired sleep, impaired concentration, anxiety, overeating with weight gain, anhedonia, and decreased libido. She adds that she has experienced similar symptoms each year from October through May over the last four years since relocating to the midwestern United States. Prior to 5 years ago, the patient resided in the southwestern United States and was asymptomatic.

11. Which of the following best describes this patient's DSM–IV diagnosis?

    A. major depressive disorder (single episode, severe)

    B. adjustment disorder with depressed mood (chronic)

    C. major depressive disorder, (recurrent, severe, with seasonal pattern)

    D. bipolar II disorder, (depressed, severe, with seasonal pattern)

    E. posttraumatic stress disorder, (chronic, with delayed onset)

12. Which of the following medications would MOST appropriately treat symptoms of this patient?
   A. alprazolam
   B. sertraline
   C. lithium carbonate
   D. benztropine
   E. haloperidol

13. After six weeks of treatment with the medication chosen in question 12, the patient has experienced a slight improvement, but severe depressive symptoms persist. Which of the following treatment modalities would be your FIRST choice as adjunctive treatment to her medication?
   A. electroconvulsive therapy
   B. psychoanalysis
   C. psychostimulant therapy
   D. psychosurgery
   E. phototherapy

Questions 14 through 17

A 45-year-old divorced woman is self-referred for psychiatric services. She complains of depressed mood for 4 to 5 months. This is accompanied by anger, irritability, poor appetite with weight loss, social isolation, tearfulness, poor concentration, impaired sleep, and suicidal ideation. Past psychiatric history is significant for a 6-month course of marital therapy. Current psychosocial stressors include financial pressures and conflicts in her relationship with a significant other.

14. Which of the following BEST describes this patient's DSM–IV diagnosis?
   A. borderline personality disorder
   B. major depressive disorder (single episode, severe, without psychotic features)
   C. adjustment disorder with mixed anxiety and depressed mood
   D. histrionic personality disorder
   E. bipolar II disorder (depressed, severe)

15. Which of the following medications would MOST appropriately treat the symptoms of this patient?

    A. fluoxetine
    B. carbamazepine
    C. diphenhydramine
    D. fluphenazine
    E. risperidone

16. After 4 weeks of treatment with the medication chosen in question 15, the patient reports improvement in all of her symptoms. She adds that she and her significant other are getting along much better, as well. She is concerned, however, because she has experienced some decreased interest in sex and anorgasmia. What is the MOST likely cause of her new complaint?

    A. a previously unrecognized sexual dysfunction disorder
    B. severe interpersonal conflict with her significant other
    C. a manifestation of her underlying personality disorder
    D. a side effect from the medication chosen in question 15
    E. a factitious complaint in keeping with her attention-seeking behavior pattern

17. What is the MOST appropriate treatment at this point?

    A. decrease the medication dosage and schedule follow-up appointment
    B. referral for couple's counseling
    C. referral to sexual disorders clinic
    D. confrontation regarding the attention seeking behavior
    E. referral for electroconvulsive therapy

Questions 18 through 22

A 19-year-old woman is attempting to gain entrance to the White House to speak with the President of the United States. She states that she wishes to complain about mental health care in this country. She has threatened to harm White House staff, Secret Service personnel, and others for preventing her from seeing the President. When you examine her, she speaks rapidly and with pressured speech. She discusses, at length, her special powers and the fact that God speaks to her directly. Her family adds that she has not slept in several nights and that she has serious financial problems due to excessive use of her credit cards.

18. Which of the following DSM–IV diagnoses BEST describes this patient's condition?
   A. bipolar I disorder (single manic episode, severe with mood congruent psychotic features)
   B. bipolar II disorder (most recent episode hypomanic, severe, with psychotic features)
   C. posttraumatic stress disorder
   D. adjustment disorder with disturbance of conduct
   E. intermittent explosive disorder

19. Which of the following medication combinations would be the MOST useful in treating this patient?
   A. lithium carbonate/amitriptyline
   B. lithium carbonate/aminophylline
   C. lithium carbonate/haloperidol
   D. paroxetine/haloperidol
   E. paroxetine/thiothixene

20. Which of the following laboratory studies would be essential to obtain prior to initiating the medications chosen in question 19?
   A. CAT scan of head
   B. EEG
   C. liver panel
   D. pregnancy test
   E. vitamin B_{12} level

21. A few hours after initiation of the therapy chosen in question 19, the patient complains of severe eye pain, and eyes are noted to be "locked" in an elevated position. These symptoms are called
    A. akathisia
    B. acute dystonic reaction
    C. parkinsonian syndrome
    D. tardive dyskinesia
    E. anticholinergic effect

22. Which of the following is the MOST appropriate treatment of the condition described in question 21?
    A. haloperidol, 10 mg IM
    B. haloperidol, 10 mg IV
    C. benztropine, 2.0 mg PO
    D. diphenhydramine, 50 mg IV
    E. amantadine, 100 mg PO

Questions 23 and 24

A 27-year-old divorced elementary schoolteacher is coerced into psychiatric consultation by her mother. She states that her mother does not believe that a prominent major league baseball player is in love with her. She states that this relationship has been going on when she attended the baseball player's autograph signing party at a local mall since 2 years ago. Although they do not communicate directly, she watches his televised baseball games faithfully because he often uses baseball signals to communicate special messages to her. Her work is going well, although she has recently begun using her sick days to attend afternoon baseball games. Her home life is unremarkable except that the patient often neglects household tasks due to her extensive watching of televised baseball games. A physical examination and routine laboratory work are reported to be normal.

23. Which of the following BEST describes the patient's DSM–IV diagnosis?
    A. delusional disorder (grandiose type)
    B. schizophrenia (undifferentiated type)
    C. bipolar II disorder (most recent episode hypomanic)
    D. delusional disorder (erotomanic type)
    E. delusional disorder (jealous type)

24. The MOST effective psychotherapeutic approach to this patient is to
   A. pretend to give credence to her delusional beliefs
   B. develop a paternalistic approach
   C. attempt to talk the patient out of her delusional beliefs, with logical reasoning
   D. confront the patient with the evidence that refutes the validity of her beliefs
   E. convey that you do not accept her beliefs, but make it clear that this disagreement implies no disrespect

Questions 25 and 26

A 64-year-old widowed male is referred for psychiatric evaluation by his dermatologist. He complains of a skin condition that has been present for seven years. He states that his skin has been infested by an unusual microorganism that is related to the organism which causes tuberculosis. He has seen numerous dermatologists over the years in the hopes that someone would make the correct diagnosis and would prescribe antituberculosis medications. Meanwhile, he complains of extensive loss of head and facial hair due to this condition and considerable itching. Because he believes that the infestation is highly contagious, the patient has discontinued contact with his grandchildren, friends, and other relatives. A recent medical evaluation revealed mild hypertension but was otherwise unremarkable.

25. Which of the following BEST describes this patient's DSM–IV diagnosis?
   A. schizophreniform disorder
   B. delusional disorder (somatic type)
   C. delusional disorder (persecutory type)
   D. paranoid personality disorder
   E. panic disorder with agoraphobia

26. Which of the following medications is MOST likely to be effective in treating this patient?
   A. sertraline
   B. nortriptyline
   C. carbamazepine
   D. pimozide
   E. alprazolam

Questions 27 through 30

A 68-year-old married woman is referred for psychiatric evaluation by her family physician. She complains of 10 months of "anxiety episodes," which are characterized by hyperventilation, feeling cold, chest tightness, difficulty breathing, sweating, and intense fear. The first episode occurred while she was awaiting an MRI scan to evaluate a knee injury. Since then, these events have occurred several times each week—generally upon awakening in the morning and occasionally while at work. The patient has begun to greatly fear having an episode while at work. She is also afraid to go to sleep at night due to fear of awakening with one of these episodes.

27. Which of the following DSM–IV diagnoses BEST describes this patient's symptoms?
    A. panic disorder with agoraphobia
    B. panic disorder without agoraphobia
    C. generalized anxiety disorder
    D. posttraumatic stress disorder
    E. adjustment disorder with anxiety

28. Which of the following medications would BEST treat this patient?
    A. alprazolam
    B. diazepam
    C. haloperidol
    D. risperidone
    E. clozapine

29. Which of the following medications might you choose if you learned that this patient also had a diagnosis of alcohol dependence?
    A. lorazepam
    B. diazepam
    C. alprazolam
    D. imipramine
    E. thiothixene

30. Which of the following psychotherapeutic measures may be helpful for this patient?

    A. cognitive therapy to identify distorted patterns of thinking

    B. assertiveness training

    C. psychoeducation

    D. group therapy

    E. all of the above

Questions 31 through 33

A 39-year-old married mother of two presents for psychiatric treatment, stating, "My rituals are taking over my life." She reports being afraid that she or her sons will die if activities are not carried out in the "proper way." For her, this means repeating all household tasks three times. In addition, certain chants must be repeated numerous times throughout the day in order to keep her children safe. Certain items, such as old clothing or towels are not discarded for fear that "something terrible will happen." She states that these rituals have consumed all of her time, such that she is no longer able to work or socialize.

31. Which of the following DSM–IV diagnoses MOST accurately describes this patient's symptoms?

    A. generalized anxiety disorder

    B. anxiety disorder, NOS

    C. obsessive/compulsive disorder

    D. panic disorder with agoraphobia

    E. adjustment disorder with anxiety

32. Which one of the following medications would be the most effective choice to treat this patient?

    A. alprazolam

    B. amitriptyline

    C. clozaril

    D. clomipramine

    E. imipramine

33. If the medication chosen in question 32 was not effective, which
of the following medications would be an effective alternative?

A. diazepam

B. fluoxetine

C. fluphenazine

D. buspirone

E. trifluoperazine

Questions 34 through 40

An agitated 24-year-old unmarried white man is brought to the emergency room by the police. He has a five-year history of multiple-drug
abuse. He does not work and lives with people he meets on the streets.
In the past, he has supported himself through drug dealing and shoplift-
ing. He reports having no friends.

About five years ago, he began to develop feelings of vague suspiciousness. He recognized that this was just his way of perceiving the
world, rather than reality. However, three days ago his suspiciousness
increased. He now has trouble sleeping. He has become convinced that
his neighbor is a member of the Mafia and is plotting to kill him. This
evening, he went to his neighbor's house in an attempt to eavesdrop.
The neighbor saw him and came to the door. The patient shot him.

34. The axis IV diagnosis is

A. none

B. threat of job loss

C. partner relational problem

D. unemployment and homelessness

E. illiteracy

35. For current global assessment of functioning (GAF), the axis V
diagnosis is

A. 70

B. 20

C. 40

D. 50

E. 0

36. The axis I differential diagnosis does NOT include
   A. alcohol-induced psychotic disorder
   B. amphetamine-induced psychotic disorder
   C. amphetamine intoxication
   D. schizophrenic disorder (paranoid)
   E. dysthymic disorder

37. If this syndrome were alcoholic hallucinosis, the clinical history would include
   A. auditory hallucinations
   B. clouding of consciousness
   C. "rum fits"
   D. family history of alcoholism
   E. prominent paranoid delusions

38. If this syndrome were amphetamine-induced psychotic disorder with delusions, the clinical history would likely include
   A. aggressiveness and hostility
   B. visual hallucinations
   C. psychomotor retardation
   D. bulimia
   E. strephosymbolia

39. The immediate treatment of choice for this person includes
   A. insight-oriented therapy
   B. antipsychotic and supportive therapy
   C. barbiturates
   D. ECT
   E. methadone

40. This patient's attorney could argue that his client is not legally responsible for shooting his neighbor because
   A. he was suffering from a substance-induced psychotic disorder at the time
   B. the neighbor was, in fact, a member of the Mafia
   C. he is incompetent to stand trial
   D. he didn't know the gun was loaded
   E. none of the above

Questions 41 through 43

A 22-year-old single man presents to the psychiatric crisis service because he "doesn't know what else to do." He relates that about one year ago he began to hear voices talking to him, telling him things about people around him. At other times, he is able to hear people around him talking about him, even though he knows that they are too far away for him to actually be hearing them.

He is presently in his third year of a five-year plumbing apprenticeship. He is having difficulty at work—his foreman has noticed his difficulty concentrating, distractibility, and frequent mistakes. He became particularly concerned after camping outdoors two nights ago and experiencing auditory and visual hallucinations, accompanied by the strong feeling that someone was going to sneak up and kill him. He sheepishly admits that he had been drinking quite a few beers and had smoked a joint. He says that this is only the second time he has ever used marijuana; the first was some 3 to 4 years ago.

41. Diagnostic possibilities would include all of the following EXCEPT
   A. major depression with psychotic features
   B. paranoid schizophrenia
   C. shared psychotic disorder
   D. schizoaffective disorder
   E. atypical psychosis

42. To meet the criteria for major depression with psychotic features, which of the following must be TRUE?
   A. the delusions and hallucinations involve typical depressive themes of personal inadequacy, guilt, death, and punishment
   B. the patient has experienced either depressed mood or anhedonia
   C. symptoms of depression began at least two weeks before the onset of hallucinations
   D. patient has experienced recurrent suicidal ideation
   E. none of the above

43. Symptoms that the patient has described include
   A. loose association
   B. depersonalization
   C. cannabis abuse
   D. auditory hallucinations
   E. derailment

Questions 44 and 45

A 27-year-old man comes to your office seeking help for his compulsive masturbation. He relates that on a daily basis he feels the overwhelming urge to masturbate into a high-heeled shoe that he kept as a memento from a previous relationship. He says that this has been going on for the past three years and is causing difficulties in his current relationship. Recently the strife in his current relationship has caused him to feel sad most days with some increased sleep latency and lack of interest in normally pleasurable activities. He denies any other depressive or anxious symptomatology.

44. His sexual disorder is BEST characterized diagnostically as
   A. dyspareunia
   B. pedophilia
   C. frotteurism
   D. fetishism
   E. exhibitionism

45. His mood symptomatology is BEST characterized diagnostically as
   A. major depression (single, mild)
   B. dysthymic disorder
   C. depressive disorder due to sexual dysfunction
   D. adjustment disorder with depressed mood
   E. cyclothymic disorder

Question 46

46. A 62-year-old woman is referred to you by her attorney to ensure that she is competent to make out her will. She is rather wealthy and has Alzheimer's disease that is progressing steadily. In order to ascertain her testamentary capacity, you must assess all of the following EXCEPT

    A. her knowledge regarding the nature and extent of her property

    B. her understanding of the nature of making a bequest

    C. her ability to perform simple calculations

    D. her knowledge of her natural beneficiaries

Questions 47 through 49

A 43-year-old unemployed, undomiciled, man is admitted to your inpatient unit voluntarily. He voices complaints of suicidal ideation and says, "I'll do it if you don't help me." He offers no physical complaints beyond a frontal headache. He denies substance abuse/dependence and any prior history of psychiatric illness. He tells all this to the admitting physician, but when he reaches your unit, he scowls and says, "I'm not answering any more damn questions," and disengages. Without verbal stimulations, he falls soundly asleep in front of the televisions. When watching the televisions, he consults the weekly *T.V. Guide* and selects programs he wants to watch. At no time does he appear to be agitated or responding to internal stimuli. He is social with other patients. He ate ravenously when awake.

His admission physical shows him to be afebrile with a regular pulse of 104/min, blood pressure 180/110, and respiratory rate of 18/min. He was not ataxic and did not exhibit hand or tongue tremors. His pupils were dilated. There were no focal neurological signs. His blood alcohol was zero. Complete blood count, electrolytes, and liver function tests were within normal limits. His ECG showed a sinus tachycardia.

    47. Which of the following diagnoses is MOST likely given his presentation?

        A. Wernicke's encephalopathy

        B. schizophrenic exacerbation

        C. major depression with suicidal intent

        D. cocaine intoxication and withdrawal

        E. a panic attack

48. You now receive a call from a family member who tells you that the patient has been in six area drug treatment programs, was just in a hospital across town, and is wanted for a serious assault by the police. What diagnosis would you now consider as the MOST likely addition to your first one?
   A. antisocial personality disorder
   B. psychosis, NOS
   C. narcissistic personality disorder
   D. paranoid personality disorder
   E. borderline personality disorder

49. Which statement does NOT describe an expected clinical course in treating this patient, given his presentation?
   A. unrelenting claims of suicidal thoughts in the face of a responsive mood, normal energy level, and appetite
   B. cooperation with ward policies and routine
   C. a urine drug screen positive for cocaine and benzodiazepines
   D. a postintoxication depression
   E. no serious ongoing physical sequelae

Questions 50 through 53

Since she was 8 years old, a 28-year-old woman has had difficulties talking in class, participating in group discussion, and giving speeches. Despite this, she has risen to middle management at an accounting firm and is known as a good worker. She has no symptoms of anxiety outside of the above situations. There is no history of prior psychological assessment or therapy. She denies a history of alcohol and drug abuse. There is no history of medical illness, and she takes no prescribed medications. She has a close circle of steady friends. Her father is described as shy and anxious.

Her main complaint is that she finds herself avoiding meetings that could help with job advancement because, "I can't sleep or think if I know I have to go to one." When she does attend, she states that her voice wavers, her hands tremble, and she feels her heart racing.

50. Which of the following diagnoses is MOST likely in this case?
    A. panic attacks
    B. social phobia
    C. specific phobia
    D. panic attacks with agoraphobia
    E. schizoid personality disorder

51. The lifetime prevalence of social phobia from epidemiological and community-based studies has a range of
    A. 0.5% to 1%
    B. 1% to 3%
    C. 3% to 13%
    D. 10% to 20%
    E. 20% to 30%

52. All ot the following statements about social phobia are true EXCEPT
    A. typical onset is in the mid-teens
    B. the usual course is for it to remit in young adulthood
    C. often there is a childhood history of social inhibition or shyness
    D. onset can abruptly follow a stressful or humiliating experience
    E. severity may fluctuate with life stressors and demands

53. Treatments for social phobias include all of the following EXCEPT
- **A.** monoamine oxidase inhibitors
- **B.** propranolol
- **C.** clonazepam
- **D.** desensitization
- **E.** analytical psychotherapy

Questions 54 through 56

A 35-year-old divorced mother of two is admitted to your acute inpatient psychiatry unit with first-time complaints of depressions and thoughts of suicide. By report, she was in a singles bar the night before and approached an undercover male police officer and, in the course of their conversation, she invited him to her house to "tie her up." When the officer said, "How much?," she answered, "We'll see how much." He then arrested her for soliciting. She swears she was talking about "how much" she would let him tie her up.

She has no criminal record and no history of psychiatric illness. There is no history of alcohol and drug abuse. By all accounts, she is an excellent mother and a valued employee at a local restaurant.

54. If you accept that she is telling the truth, what is the MOST likely diagnosis?
- **A.** paraphilia
- **B.** borderline personality disorder
- **C.** bipolar disorder (manic phase)
- **D.** antisocial personality disorder
- **E.** major depression

55. Sexual masochism includes all of the following behaviors EXCEPT
- **A.** blindfolding
- **B.** paddling, spanking, or whipping
- **C.** cross-dressing
- **D.** pinning and piercing
- **E.** rubbing a nonconsenting person

56. The condition in question 54 includes all of the following EXCEPT

    A. exhibitionism

    B. voyeurism

    C. pedophilia

    D. homosexuality

    E. fetishism

Questions 57 and 58

A 25-year-old woman seeks psychiatric help for depression related to marital conflicts. Her husband accuses her of "acting like a tramp" and is threatening to leave her. She is now feeling suicidal and has considered combining "all sorts of pills" and alcohol as a way to do it. She acknowledges having tried this on at least four other occasions. She does admit to "bar-hopping" with girlfriends and regularly becomes "tipsy." She admits to not always knowing how she gets home from the bar. She expresses concern that the alcohol does "numb-out" the "humming and whispering in my mind" which alerts her "to trouble." She calls it "my little signal from heaven" and laughs (rather delightfully and infectiously), saying, "I bet you think I'm crazy!"

57. Of the following, the LEAST likely diagnosis is

    A. bipolar II disorder

    B. bipolar I disorder

    C. histrionic personality disorder

    D. obsessive–compulsive personality disorder

    E. borderline personality disorder

58. All of the following are high-risk factors for suicide in the woman except

    A. alcohol abuse

    B. prior suicidal behavior

    C. emotional lability or extremes

    D. married

    E. conflictual marital relationship

Questions 59 and 60

The same woman (in questions 57 through 62) describes her life before age 22 as "normal." She completed high school in the upper 25% of her class. Completed a degree in fine arts and began to teach in a local high school She describes her relationships with her parents as "warm and close," denies any early sexual behaviors in her teen years, and says she had "many friends, boys and girls, some close, some not so close." She denies any problems with the law, alcohol, or drug use prior to age 23.

59. The most likely diagnosis at this time is
    A. bipolar II disorder
    B. histrionic personality disorder
    C. borderline personality disorder
    D. adjustment disorder
    E. none of the above

60. Which of the following (if found) could explain the woman's symptoms and behaviors?
    A. history of rape
    B. hyperthyroidism
    C. pernicious anemia
    D. all of the above
    E. none of the above

Directions (Questions 61 through 66): Each of the questions or incomplete statements below is followed by five suggested answers or completions. Select the ONE that is best in each case.

---

61. A 3-year-old child presents with her parents, who are concerned that she continues to wet her bed nightly. While she has mastered toilet training during the daytime for approximately the past 6 months, she has yet to have a dry night. She has no symptoms of burning or frequency. You should

  A. recommend a thorough urologic evaluation by the child's pediatrician

  B. suggest the use of a bell and pad to behaviorally train the child

  C. question the parents about family stressors

  D. reassure the parents that this is the normal progression of sphincter control

  E. prescribe imipramine

62. A 4-year-old boy presents with his parents, who describe long-standing significant difficulties with peer relationships in preschool and the neighborhood. They state that he likes to be alone, rarely seeking out even his parents for contact. He seems very interested in carefully aligning blocks while waving his arms in an unusual way or in running the vacuum cleaner. What developmental line would be most helpful to ask about at this point?

  A. gender identity

  B. moral reasoning

  C. language development

  D. ability to understand cause and effect relationships

  E. sleep history

63. A 9-year-old boy presents to your office on referral by his pediatrician because of a history of inattentiveness, impulsivity, hyperactivity, and aggressiveness, both at home and at school. His parents request that you do "a test" to determine if he has attention-deficit hyperactivity disorder (ADHD). You

  A. order an EEG

  B. order a PET scan

    C. check endogenous stimulant levels

    D. collect additional history

    E. order a Wechsler Intelligence Scale for Children (WISC)

64. Upon gathering further data from the patient, family, and school, you diagnose the patient as having ADHD, but you also note during your exam that the boy frequently blinks and clears his throat. Should you elect to treat him with medication, you should consider

    A. stimulant medications are likely to exacerbate a tic disorder

    B. reports have been made concerning a risk of sudden death with tricyclic antidepressants (TCAs) in children

    C. clonidine has been reported efficacious in the treatment of Tourette's syndrome

    D. the precise mechanism of action of stimulants is unknown

    E. all of the above

65. A patient has had psychotherapy to address his difficulties at work dealing with his boss. After several sessions, he decides to begin psychoanalysis to better understand himself. The following statements about psychoanalysis are true EXCEPT

    A. it could last 3 to 6 years, 4 to 5 times per week

    B. it examines the relationship with the analyst

    C. it views the patient's conscious thoughts as central to current symptoms

    D. it focuses on recovering early life conflicts and their consequences in adult life

    E. it requires neutrality on the part of the analyst

66. Other forms of psychotherapy that may include psychoanalytic principals include all of the following EXCEPT

    A. brief psychodynamic psychotherapy

    B. group psychotherapy

    C. systematic desensitization

    D. explorative psychotherapy

    E. supportive psychotherapy

Case Studies

Explanatory Answers

1. (E) Hypoglycemia can often present with hallucinations and agitation, as well as sweating and tremor. Alcohol withdrawal can also cause many of those symptoms. Phantom limb syndrome occurs in individuals who have had an amputation who still seem to feel the amputated limb's presence; it does not appear immediately relevant for this patient. (**Ref. 1,** pp. 372, 772; **Ref. 5,** p. 40)

2. (A) A STAT glucose is likely to show hypoglycemia in this patient, who has insulin-dependent diabetes mellitus. She likely is experiencing a hypoglycemic episode. (**Ref. 1,** pp. 372, 772)

3. (B) This woman is most likely suffering from a hypoglycemic episode. She needs to have her glucose restored to a normal level to prevent permanent brain damage. If it turns out that there is some other cause of her hallucinations, the administration of the glucose will not cause permanent harm and can be handled by adjusting her insulin dosages. (**Ref. 1,** pp. 372, 772)

4. (B) This patient may be experiencing a manic episode. An increase in sexual desire, reckless spending, and even auditory hallucinations are common in mania. A history of similar episodes would be very useful in making the differential diagnosis between a manic episode and another psychotic disorder. The history of an appendectomy in the patient is largely irrelevant. (**Ref. 6,** pp. 196–200)

5. (**C**) Antipsychotic medication is often needed for the immediate relief of severe agitation and psychosis in a manic patient and to allow the patient to sleep. Haloperidol is a good choice. Lithium carbonate, valproic acid, and carbamazepine are all antimanic drugs which take several days to take effect, while amitriptyline is a tricyclic antidepressant and can induce rapid cycling in bipolar I disorder patient treated with it. (**Ref. 1,** pp. 553–554)

6. (**C**) The most common guidelines for the treatment of acute mania are for lithium blood levels of 1.0 to 1.5 mEq/L; 0.6 to 1.2 mEq/L is a typical recommended dose for maintenance treatment of individuals with bipolar I disorder. Serious toxicity is likely to occur with lithium levels higher than 3.0 mEq/L, and, sometimes, at slightly lower doses, depending on the patient. (**Ref. 1,** pp. 961–969)

7. (**D**) Tremor occurs in the hands of many patients on therapeutic doses of lithium. Lithium can cause renal problems, including decreased creatinine clearance and decreased urine concentrating ability, and it can cause hypothyroidism in 7% to 9% of patients on long-term lithium treatment. There is no known relationship of lithium treatment to the malignant transformation of a skin mole, but psoriasis is a possible dermatological side effect of lithium treatment. (**Ref. 1,** pp. 961–969)

8. (**B**) Each of the listed questions is likely to be useful in the evaluation of this patient, who may suffer from borderline personality disorder. Because of the urgency of the problem, however, the degree of suicidality or homicidality of the patient is the most important immediate question to ask the patient, and it should be asked directly. (**Ref. 3,** pp. 28, 187–188)

9. (**D**) Individuals with borderline personality disorder tend to perceive people and objects as all good or all bad. They are likely to engage in self-destructive behavior, including sexual acting out. It is important for the staff to communicate closely on the treatment of such patients to prevent their being played against each other by the patient. Involuntary urinary incontinence is not a typical

feature of borderline personality disorder in a patient who does not have some other explanation for the incontinence. (**Ref. 1,** pp. 739–741; **Ref. 3,** pp. 187–188)

10. **(D)** Patients with borderline personality disorder usually gain greater stability in relationships and vocational functioning during their 30s, 40s, and thereafter. There is not usually a progression toward schizophrenia, but there is a high incidence of episodes of major depressive disorder and of self-harm in these patients. (**Ref. 1,** pp. 739–741; **Ref. 4,** pp. 652–653)

11. **(C)** The patient described meets the criteria for major depressive episode, based on symptoms of depressed mood, diminished interest or pleasure in activities, increased appetite with weight gain, and disturbance of sleep for greater than a two-week period. In addition, there has been a regular temporal relationship between the onset of major depressive episode and a particular time of the year for more than two years. Therefore, patient's presentation best meets criteria for a major depressive disorder (recurrent, severe, with seasonal pattern). (**Ref. 3,** pp. 201–204; **Ref. 4,** pp. 327, 390).

12. **(B)** Alprazolam is an anxiolytic medication in the benzodiazepine group. Sertraline is an antidepressant medication in the selective serotonin reuptake inhibitor group. Lithium carbonate is a mood-stabilizing agent that also has some antidepressant properties. Benztropine is an anticholinergic medication useful in managing neuroleptic side effects. Haloperidol is an antipsychotic medication in the butyrophenone category. Of these choices, sertraline is the most appropriate medication for this patient. (**Ref. 3,** pp. 160, 164, 217–223)

13. **(E)** Electroconvulsive therapy is a good choice for patients who cannot tolerate side effects of antidepressant medications, patients with refractory depressions, and elderly depressed patients. The goal of psychoanalysis is resolution of symptoms and major reworking of personality structures related to childhood conflicts. Psychostimulant medications are used in treatment of depressed medical patients who cannot tolerate other antidepressant medications. Psychosurgical techniques have been beneficial in severe, debilitating cases of obsessive-compulsive disorder that have

failed other types of treatment. In some patients with the condition described in question 11, phototherapy or light therapy has been a useful adjunct and even replacement to medication therapy. (**Ref. 3**, pp. 217–223, 259, 481–484)

14. **(B)** The patient described meets the criteria for major depressive episode, based on symptoms of depressed mood, decreased appetite with weight loss, disturbed sleep, impaired concentration, and suicidal ideation for greater than a two-week period. This is the first major depressive episode known for this patient. Several symptoms in excess of those required to make the diagnosis are present. Therefore, the patient's presentation best meets the criteria for major depressive disorder (single episode, severe, without psychotic features). (**Ref. 3**, pp. 201–204; **Ref. 4**, pp. 327, 344, 378)

15. **(A)** Fluoxetine is an antidepressant medication in the selective serotonin reuptake inhibitor group. Carbamazepine is a mood-stabilizing and anticonvulsant medication. Diphenhydramine is an antihistamine with anticholinergic properties, useful in managing neuroleptic side effects. Fluphenazine and risperidone are antipsychotic medications. Of these choices, fluoxetine is the most appropriate medication for this patient. (**Ref. 3**, pp. 217–223, 160, 164)

16. **(D)** Sexual difficulties, including delayed ejaculation in men and anorgasmia in both men and women, have been reported as side effects from fluoxetine therapy. Oftentimes, patients will not spontaneously report these problems, and it is incumbent upon the therapist to inquire about them. (**Ref. 3**, pp. 523–526)

17. **(A)** At times, the sexual side effects occurring with fluoxetine will resolve with a reduced dosage. Since the patient has otherwise had a good response to this medication, it would be logical to try this step first. (**Ref. 3**, pp. 521–526)

18. **(A)** The patient described meets the criteria for a manic episode, based on a persistent elevated, expansive, or irritable mood, along with grandiosity, decreased need for sleep, talkativeness with pressured speech, and excessive involvement in pleasurable activities. Since there is no known history of previous manic episodes,

this condition would be called bipolar I disorder (single manic episode). Since psychotic features are present which follow a typical manic theme of special relationship to a deity or famous person, the complete diagnosis would be bipolar I disorder (single manic episode, severe, with mood-congruent psychotic features). (**Ref. 3,** pp. 211–214; **Ref. 4,** pp. 332, 355, 379–380)

19. **(C)** Lithium carbonate is a mood-stabilizing agent. Amitriptyline is an antidepressant medication in the tricyclic group. Aminophylline is a bronchodilator medication. Haloperidol is an antipsychotic medication in the butyrophenone category. Paroxetine is an antidepressant medication in the selective serotonin reuptake inhibitor group. Thiothixene is an antipsychotic medication in the thioxanthene category. Since this patient demonstrates both mood and psychotic symptoms, the most effective treatment would be a mood-stabilizing agent, plus an antipsychotic agent. Generally, the antipsychotic medication may be discontinued once the patient has been stabilized. (**Ref. 3,** pp. 160, 217–224)

20. **(D)** Lithium can cause severe fetal cardiovascular abnormalities if taken during the first trimester of pregnancy. Thus, obtaining a prelithium pregnancy test is essential in all premenopausal females. (**Ref. 3,** pp. 223–224)

21. **(B)** Akathisia is an unpleasant feeling of restlessness and the inability to sit still. Parkinsonian syndrome includes masked facies, cogwheel rigidity, bradykinesia, and "pill-rolling" tremor. Tardive dyskinesia is characterized by involuntary movements of the face, trunk, or extremities. Anticholinergic effects include dry mouth, decreased sweating, decreased bronchial secretions, blurred vision, urinary retention, and constipation. Acute dystonic reactions are frightening and disturbing reactions that most frequently occur within hours or days of the initiation of antipsychiatric therapy. The most common features include uncontrollable tightening and spasm of face, neck, head, back, or extraocular muscles. (**Ref. 3,** pp. 512–518).

22. **(D)** Haloperidol is an antipsychotic medication in the butyrophenone category. Intramuscular or intravenous administration of haloperidol could worsen this condition. Benztropine is an anticholinergic medication and could effectively treat this condition.

However, oral administration would not provide rapid enough relief of the acute pain symptoms. Amantadine is a dopamine-agonist medication, useful in the treatment of some extrapyramidal disorders. Diphenhydramine is an antihistamine with anticholinergic properties. Intravenous administration of anticholinergic medication is necessary to provide rapid relief of acute dystonic reactions. (**Ref. 3,** pp. 512–518)

23. **(D)** The patient described best meets the criteria for delusional disorder, based on symptoms of a nonbizarre delusion of greater than one month's duration and functioning that is not markedly impaired apart from the impact of the delusion. Patients who have delusions that another person, usually of higher status, is in love with them are assigned the specific erotomanic type. Therefore, this patient's presentation best meets the criteria for delusional disorder (erotomanic type). (**Ref. 2,** pp. 219–220, **Ref. 4,** p. 301)

24. **(E)** In treating the patient with delusional disorder, complete frankness is necessary. The clinician should make it clear that delusional beliefs are not accepted but that disagreement implies no disrespect. (**Ref. 2,** pp. 221–222)

25. **(B)** The patient described best meets criteria for delusional disorder, based on symptoms of a nonbizarre delusion of greater than one month's duration and functioning that is not markedly impaired apart from the impact of the delusion or its ramifications. Patients who have delusions that they have some physical defect or general medical condition are assigned to the specifier "somatic type." Therefore, this patient's presentation best meets criteria for delusional disorder (somatic type). In the past, this condition has also been called monosymptomatic hypochondriasis. (**Ref. 2,** pp. 219–220, **Ref. 4,** p. 301)

26. **(D)** Sertraline is an antidepressant medication in the selective serotonin reuptake inhibitor group. Nortriptyline is an antidepressant medication in the tricyclic group. Carbamazepine is a mood stabilizing and anticonvulsant medication. Alprazolam is an anxiolytic medication in the benzodiazepine group. Pimozide is an antipsychotic medication in the diphenylbutylpiperidine group. Of the medications listed, pimozide appears to have some specific ef-

ficacy in patients with delusions of infestation. (**Ref. 2,** pp. 221–222; **Ref. 3,** p. 160)

27. **(B)** The patient described suffers from panic attacks, which are a discrete period of intense fear with associated physical symptoms of difficulty breathing, chills, chest discomfort, and sweating. Since she has persistent concerns about having additional attacks for greater than one month, and since she does not suffer from agoraphobia, her most accurate diagnosis would be panic disorder without agoraphobia. (**Ref. 3,** pp. 234–237; **Ref. 4,** pp. 395–396, 402)

28. **(A)** Haloperidol, risperidone, and clozapine are all antipsychotic medications. Alprazolam and diazepam are benzodiazepines that are very effective in treating anxiety disorder. Diazepam is a poor choice for this patient, however, due to problems with dosage accumulation in elderly patients. Alprazolam, with specific antipanic properties, is the most appropriate medication of those listed to treat this patient's symptoms. (**Ref. 3,** pp. 240–243)

29. **(D)** Lorazepam, diazepam, and alprazolam are all benzodiazepines and would be a poor choice in patients with substance abuse problems due to their abuse potential. Thiothixene is an antipsychotic medication. Imipramine is a tricyclic antidepressant. Tricyclic antidepressants are an effective alternative treatment for panic disorder. Monoamine oxidase inhibitors and selective serotonin reuptake inhibitors may be effective alternatives as well. (**Ref. 3,** pp. 240–243)

30. **(E)** Cognitive therapy can assist patients who suffer from panic disorder in identifying distorted patterns of thinking, interrupting these thoughts and substituting either distraction or positive thoughts. Assertiveness training can help patients with symptoms of dependency, passivity, and suppressed anger, which are common in patients who suffer from panic disorder. Psychoeducation helps patients to know and to understand their diagnosis, including theories of etiology, treatment, and prognosis. Group therapy is helpful since patients benefit from recognizing that others suffer from the same disorder and from the support and encouragement of peers. (**Ref. 3,** pp. 240–243)

31. (C)   The patient described suffers from compulsions, which are repetitive behaviors that she feels driven to perform and which are aimed at preventing a dreaded event or situation. She recognizes that the compulsions are excessive or unreasonable. Her compulsions are causing marked distress, are time consuming, and are interfering with normal occupational and social functioning. Thus, the patient's presentation best meets criteria for obsessive–compulsive disorder. (**Ref. 3,** pp. 252–255; **Ref. 4,** pp. 422–423)

32. (D)   Alprazolam is an anxiolytic medication in the benzodiazepine group. Clozaril is an antipsychotic medication. Amitriptyline and imipramine are tricyclic antidepressant medications. Clomipramine is a serotonergic medication that is a specific, effective treatment for obsessive–compulsive disorder (**Ref. 3,** pp. 258–259)

33. (B)   Diazepam is an anxiolytic medication in the benzodiazepine group. Buspirone is a nonbenzodiazepine anxiolytic medication. Fluphenazine and trifluoperazine are antipsychotic medications. Fluoxetine is a specific serotonin reuptake inhibitor. These medications appear to reduce obsessive–compulsive symptoms and are a good alternative when clomipramine is not effective. (**Ref. 3,** pp. 258–259)

34. (D)   Axis IV is for reporting psychosocial and environmental problems that may affect the diagnosis, treatment, and prognosis of mental disorders. The clinician may note as many as are judged to be relevant. (**Ref. 4,** p. 29)

35. (B)   From the brief history, there is clearly some danger of his hurting himself or others, although this is not pervasive and persistent. It is important to note that this is his current GAF, and not the highest GAF for the past year. (**Ref. 4,** p. 32)

36. (E)   Given the information available, the only diagnosis not possible is dysthymic disorder; it would not account for the paranoid delusions present. (**Ref. 4,** p. 345)

37. (A)   Alcohol hallucinosis is defined as a condition of vivid auditory or visual hallucinations that develop within a few days of reduction or cessation of drinking in a physiologically dependent person. Delusions are not a prominent feature of the disorder. (**Ref. 1,** p. 408)

38. **(A)** This organic delusional syndrome develops following recent use of a sympathomimetic drug. It apparently does not develop following a single large dose unless it is preceded by chronic use. The syndrome develops rapidly. Persecutory delusions are the most prominent clinical feature. (**Ref. 1,** p. 413)

39. **(B)** The man is severely disturbed, agitated, delusional, and homicidal. Admission is crucial; treatment for the delusions should be instituted promptly. (**Ref. 1,** p. 415)

40. **(E)** In general, to be found not responsible for criminal activity, it must be determined that at the time of such conduct, as a result of mental disease or defect, he/she lacked substantial capacity either to appreciate the wrongfulness of the conduct or to conform such conduct to the requirement of the law. Usually states do not recognize substance-induced disorders as mental disease or defect. Competency to stand trial is an issue separate from criminal responsibility. (**Ref. 1,** pp. 1180–1182)

41. **(C)** Shared psychotic disorder is the development of a delusional disorder in a second person (the patient in this case) as a result of a close relationship with another person (the primary case), who already has a psychotic disorder with prominent delusions. There is no such relationship related in this case, and one of the primary symptoms—auditory hallucinations—is not part of a shared psychotic disorder. (**Ref. 1,** p. 491)

42. **(B)** For the diagnosis of major depression, either depressed mood or anhedonia must occur most of the day, nearly every day, for at least two weeks. In addition, at no time during the disturbance can there be delusions or hallucinations for as long as two weeks in the absence of prominent mood symptoms. Although not specified by DSM—IV, it would be quite unusual to have a major depression with psychotic features heralded by the psychotic components. Psychotic features may be mood congruent, but not necessarily so. (**Ref. 4,** pp. 339–345)

43. (D) The patient described auditory hallucinations, and they are a "symptom." Other choices are either not a "symptom" or were not present. (**Ref. 1,** p. 300)

44. (D) Fetishism is a type of paraphilia in which intense sexually arousing fantasies, urges, or behaviors involve nonliving objects (the "fetish"). Dyspareunia is recurrent or persistent genital pain associated with sexual intercourse. The other disorders listed are other paraphilias. (**Ref. 4,** pp. 511–513, 522–528)

45. (D) The essential feature of an adjustment disorder is the development of clinically significant emotional or behavioral symptoms in response to an identifiable stressor. This diagnosis should not be used if the disturbance meets the criteria for another axis I disorder. In this case, the mood symptomatology does not meet other axis I criteria. (**Ref. 4,** p. 623)

46. (C) Testamentary capacity refers to an individual's ability to make a will. The psychological abilities necessary to make a will are: (1) knowledge of the natural beneficiaries; (2) knowledge that they are making a bequest (will); and (3) knowledge of the nature and extent of their property (bounty). (**Ref. 1,** p. 1179)

47. (D) All things considered, this patient's presentation and subsequential course are typical for a patient who is cocaine intoxicated. He is not manifesting a delirium, nor does he have ophthalmoplegia, so Wernicke's encephalopathy is not likely. The vital sign changes are not typical of schizophrenia or major depression, nor is his objectively observed behavior. Panic attacks aren't typically hours in duration with intermittent naps. (**Ref. 1,** p. 427, 586, 817)

48. (A) With the knowledge you have, a provisional diagnostic consideration of antisocial personality disorder is most likely. There is no evidence of paranoid thought process or isolation on your unit. He has some suggestion of borderline traits with the suicidal threats but no known history of causing self-harm. One could also consider a factitious disorder with psychological signs and symptoms. (**Ref. 1,** p. 633, 738–739)

49. (B)   This patient has antisocial personality disorder complicated by cocaine withdrawal; being cooperative with staff and rules is not a typical behavior. This patient has an obvious reason to remain in the hospital with looming legal difficulties and may never deny active suicidal ideation in an effort to avoid them. **(Ref. 1,** p. 427, 633–635, 737–739, 808–811)

50. (B)   The panic symptoms as described are limited to performance situations and do not generalize beyond that. The diagnostic use of a specific phobia is limited to nonsocial and performance stimuli, such as animals, environments, and situations. Schizoid personality disorder patients would be noticeably asocial, a trait this patient does not have. **(Ref. 4,** p. 411–417)

51. (C)   The reported lifetime prevalence in the general population is 3% to 13%. Patients who present with anxiety complaints to outpatient clinics exhibit social phobia rates of 10% to 20%. **(Ref. 4,** p. 414)

52. (B)   Social phobia is frequently continuous in nature from its onset. Duration is oftentimes lifelong. The patient's level of impairment may fluctuate with exposure to the perceived stressful situations, eg, a person with social phobia may witness his fear of dating disappear when he marries and see it return if his spouse dies. **(Ref. 4,** p. 414)

53. (E)   Insight-oriented therapy is not a treatment of choice. Most clinicians stick to a combination of cognitive/behavioral techniques and the medications listed. **(Ref. 1 ,** p. 598)

54. (A)   She appears to be presenting with a paraphilia—sexual masochism, to be more precise. You have no information supporting disordered personality, nor does she meet length criteria for a mood disorder. It turns out the patient has required bondage to reach a sexual climax since her early 20s. **(Ref. 4,** p. 529)

55. (E)   There is a wide variety of masochistic behavior. Some behaviors can be life-risking, such as shocking oneself. Some may participate in oxygen-depriving activities and accidentally suffocate themselves at a reported death rate of 1 to 2 per million general population. Forced cross-dressing may be used for purposes of humiliation. Touching and rubbing someone without their consent is defined as frotteurism. (**Ref. 4,** pp. 527, 529)

56. **(D)** Homosexuality does not fit paraphilia's features, which includes intense, recurrent sexually arousing fantasies, behaviors, or sexual urges involving nonhuman objects, suffering or humiliation of oneself or one's partner or children or nonconsenting adults. Other paraphilias include frotteurism, sexual sadism, and transvestic fetishism. Paraphilias are rarely diagnosed in females. One-half of individuals who present with paraphilias are married. (**Ref. 4,** pp. 522–524)

57. **(D)** A person with obsessive–compulsive personality disorder will show emotional constriction and be preoccupied with rules and regulations. Thus far in this case, one sees a strong suggestion of affective extremes and some disregard for rules. (**Ref. 1,** p. 745)

58. **(D)** In general, being married is a low- rather than high-risk factor. In this case, it is the threat to the woman's marriage that becomes a high-risk factor. (**Ref. 1,** p. 809)

59. **(E)** The marked change in personality after age 23 suggests something other than a personality disorder occurring. The presence of a bipolar II disorder does not seem strongly supported by the initial information given. Certainly an adjustment disorder may be possible. Further investigation regarding other precipitants (trauma, medical illness, exposure to drugs, toxins, etc.) must be made before arriving at a diagnosis. (**Ref. 1,** pp. 1–5, 535–537, 728–729)

60. **(D)** A trauma such as rape may cause posttraumatic stress disorder, which may in turn precipitate both hyperthyroidism and pernicious anemia and can give rise to mania and other mood disorders. (**Ref. 1,** pp. 371, 606–611, 772–775)

61. **(D)** Control of daytime urination usually occurs by age 2-and-a-half, while lack of nighttime control generally is not a major concern until age 4. A physical exam may be helpful if physical symptoms are present or the patient was unable to master daytime sphincter control. Questioning about family stress may be indi-

cated if the child fails to progress with nighttime sphincter control. More extensive behavioral or pharmacological treatments may be considered at that time. In the meantime, encouragement, giving no fluids after supper and avoiding fluids before bed time, along with simple rewards for dry nights, will likely be successful. (**Ref. 1,** p. 45)

62. **(C)** At this point, you have data to suggest impairment in social interaction with peers and a failure to seek out parents, as well as restricted and stereotyped behaviors. This suggests a pervasive developmental disorder, and questioning about language development will help to differentiate between a diagnosis of autistic disorder and Asperger's disorder, which is characterized by a lack of significant language and cognitive delays associated with autism. (**Ref. 1,** pp. 45–47, 1052–1058, 1060–1061)

63. **(D)** There are no specific tests for ADHD. The diagnosis is a clinical one and can only be made with a careful clinical history. A differential diagnosis includes temperamental characteristics, anxiety disorder, depressive disorder, conduct disorders, and learning disorders. Conduct or learning disorders are frequently co-morbid with ADHD. Cognitive tests, such as the Continuous Performance Task, can help to confirm a diagnosis of ADHD. (**Ref. 1,** pp. 1063–1068)

64. **(D)** While stimulants, TCAs, and clonidine are all potential forms of pharmacotherapy, it may be most beneficial in this instance to initiate a trial of clonidine because it would address both symptom complexes. The guiding factor here is the level of interference of the symptoms in the child's life versus side effects of the medication. Additionally, it is important to remember that cognitive/behavioral strategies can be very successful in the treatment of symptoms of ADHD, as well as stress reduction in Tourette's disorder. (**Ref. 1,** pp. 1067, 1085)

65. **(C)** The belief that cognitions are central to producing and perpetuating symptomatology is a central tenet of cognitive psychotherapy. Psychoanalysis is founded in the belief that unconscious conflicts in an individual's past maintain themselves in the present. This is accomplished by reexperiencing and understanding past aggressive and libidinal conflicts in relation to the analyst

(the "transference neurosis"). Even though a patient must have some relative strengths to access their fantasy lives, painful neurotic conflicts can severely interfere with a person's personal life and work. (**Ref. 3,** pp. 481–484)

66. (**C**) Systematic desensitization is a behavioral approach to treating individuals with phobic problems by gradually exposing them to anxiety-provoking situations or objects in small, incremental steps. This is coupled with the teaching of relaxation responses. The remaining forms of psychotherapy listed can all utilize psychoanalytic theory in the course of treatment. (**Ref. 3,** pp. 484–487, 490–500)

References

1. Kaplan, H.I., Sadock, B.J., Grebb, J.A.: *Kaplan and Sadock's Synopsis of Psychiatry: Behavioral Sciences, Clinical Psychiatry,* ed 7. Baltimore, Williams & Wilkins, 1994.
2. Goldman, H.H.: *Review of General Psychiatry,* ed 3. Norwalk, CT, Appleton & Lange, 1992.
3. Stoudemire, A.: *Clinical Psychiatry for Medical Students,* ed 2. Philadelphia, J.B. Lippincott Company, 1994.
4. American Psychiatric Association: *Diagnostic and Statistical Manual of Mental Disorders,* ed 4. Washington, D.C., American Psychiatric Association, 1994.
5. Nicholi, A.M.: *The New Harvard Guide to Psychiatry.* Cambridge, MA, The Belknap Press of Harvard University Press, 1988.
6. Andreasen, N.C., Black, D.W.: *Introductory Textbook of Psychiatry.* Washington, D.C., American Psychiatric Press, 1991.
7. Lewis, M. *Child and Adolescent Psychiatry.* Baltimore, Williams & Wilkins, 1991.
8. Moore BE, Finz, BD. *Psychoanalytic Terms and Concepts.* New Haven, The American Psychoanalytic Association and Yale University Press, 1990.
9. Kaplan HI, Sadock BJ (eds). *Comprehensive Textbook of Psychiatry.* Vols 1, 2, ed. 5, Baltimore, Williams & Wilkins, 1989.
10. Janicak, PG, Davis JM, Preskorn, SH, Ayd, FJ. *Principles and Practice of Psychopharmacotherapy.* 1st ed, Baltimore, Williams & Wilkins, 1993.